Vitality Plan

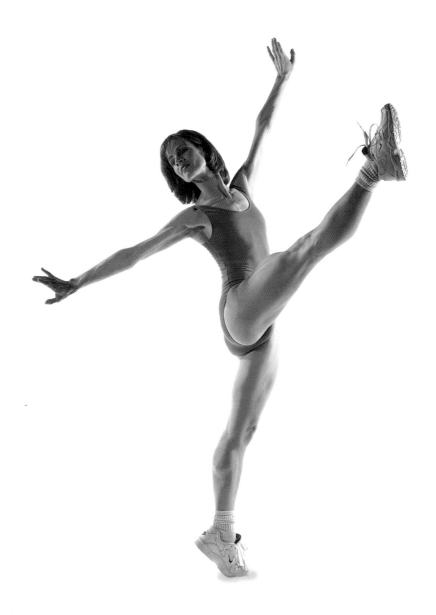

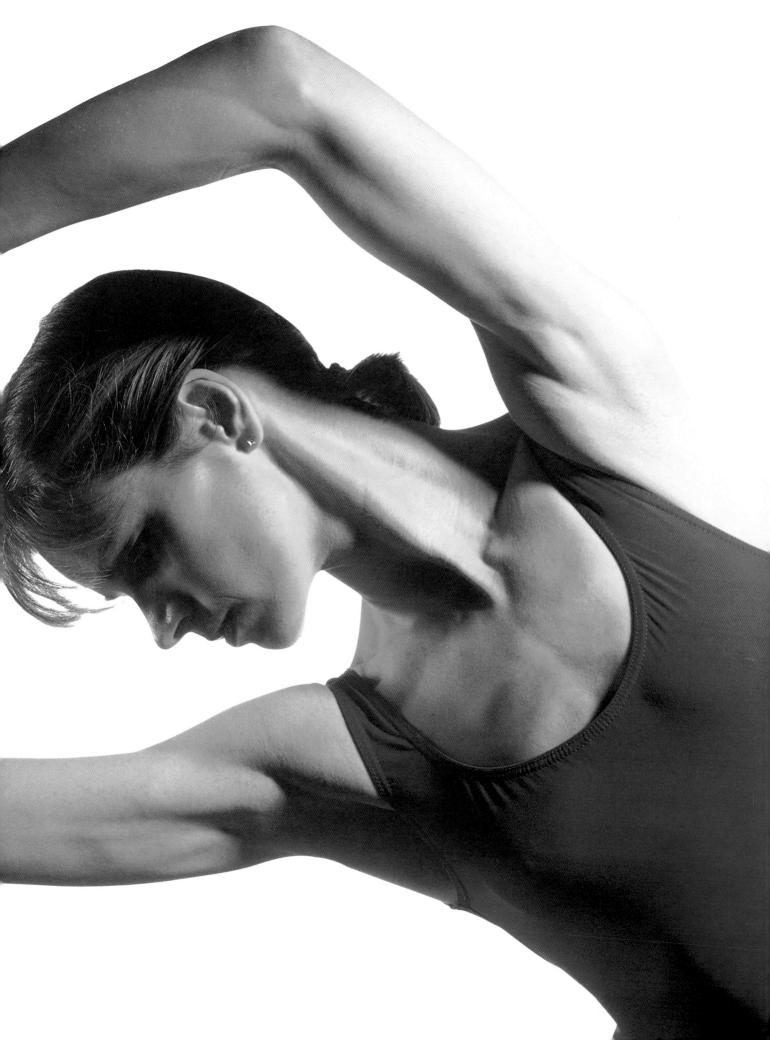

THE Vitality Plan

Deborah Bull

LONDON • NEW YORK • MOSCOW • SYDNEY

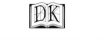

A DORLING KINDERSLEY BOOK

Project Editor Monica Chakraverty

Art Editor Robert Ford

Editor David Summers

Designer Claudia Norris

Senior Art Editor Tracey Clarke

DTP Designer Karen Ruane

Managing Editor Susannah Marriott/Mary Ling

Managing Art Editor Toni Kay

Photographers Dave King, Andy Crawford, Gary Ombler

Production Manager Maryann Rogers

"Nobody gets it wrong on purpose."
(after Socrates)

For Torje, who made sense of it all.

First published in Great Britain in 1998 by
Dorling Kindersley Limited,
9 Henrietta Street, London WC2E 8PS

Visit us on the World Wide Web at http://www.dk.com

A CIP catalogue record for this book is available
from the British Library.

ISBN 0 7513 1095 6

Reproduced in Singapore by Colourscan
Printed and bound in England by Butler and Tanner

Contents

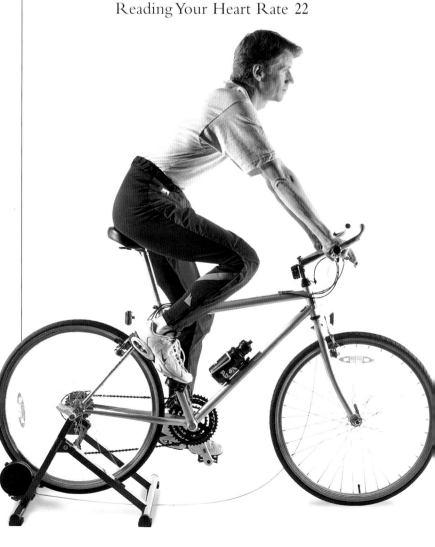

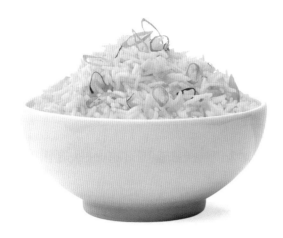

Fi

Europe is

hardly sur

become a

endure in

reached sa

The Se

The sad tr

did, the pr

not have b

it will also

As soon as

creeps bacl

You canno

a slimmer f

in a matter

right now. l

how to put

enjoying lif

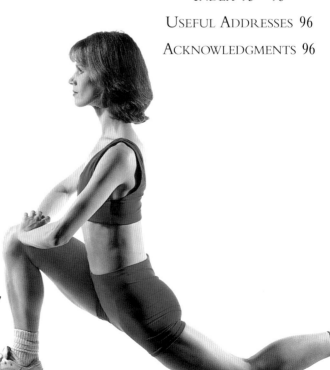

Weight Loss : The Facts

No matter how many failed diets we have under our belts, it is still

tempting to believe that there is, somewhere, a miracle diet that will help

us to shed pounds without any effort at all. I spent years searching for it, and

was taken in, time and time again, by the fresh and seductive promise of

a magic formula for weight loss.

Yet, however many diets I tried, I never managed to lose weight permanently.

It was only when I started to work with my body rather than fight against it,

that my personal battle became a thing of the past. It is the facts that provide

the answers and you need to understand those facts before weight control

makes sense. It may all seem a little complicated at first, but persevere:

battling with a few pages of information is going to

be a lot easier than battling against

your body.

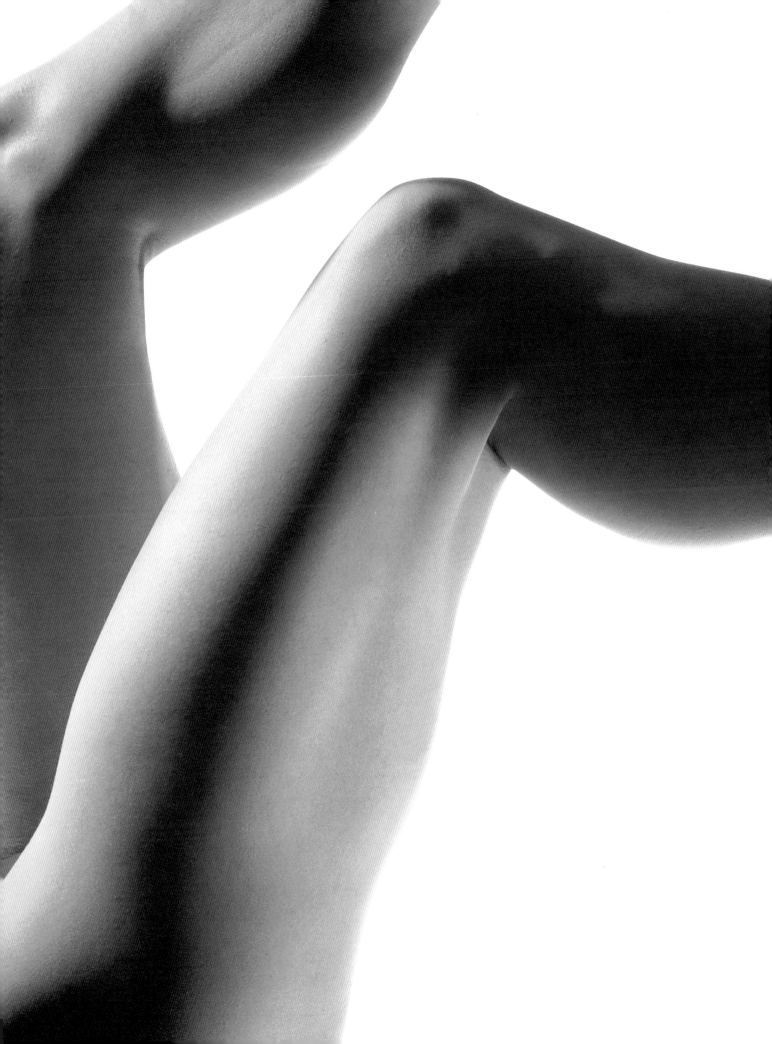

The Myths

The human body is like a machine; it operates according to certain laws that cannot be ignored. Until I understood those laws, I tried every possible way to get thin, but failed with remarkable consistency: I had the will to succeed but lacked the knowledge. But before we face the facts, let's dispel a few myths.

1 The only way to lose weight is to eat less

It is unquestionably true that you can lose weight by eating less. Everyone has done it at some point, either through choice or illness. Depriving your body of the food it needs will undoubtedly lead to rapid loss of body mass. Whether it leads to rapid loss of *fat* is another matter. It is unlikely that there is any way, apart from surgery, that fat can be lost rapidly. Furthermore, scientific research proves that weight loss through diet alone is successful in the long term less than 20% of the time – in some studies it's even less.

2 The scales never lie

Unfortunately they do. Rapid weight loss looks so good on the scales because it is mainly a loss of water and muscle. Muscle, being compact, weighs much more than fat, so two people can weigh the same yet look very different. The best way to assess progress is to:
- Throw away your scales.
- Dig out an old pair of jeans that fitted when you were happy with your body. Try them on at regular intervals until you can fasten the zip.
- Congratulate yourself and keep going.

3 If I eat less than I need, my body will have to burn its excess fat

This would seem to be logical. We all have a lot of fat stored up and it is, in some circumstances, a very efficient source of energy. Unfortunately, not in this circumstance. Your body's first priority is always to protect the brain. The brain depends on glucose, from carbohydrates, for its fuel. Fat cannot be converted into glucose but, in emergencies, when no carbohydrates are available, protein can. When starved of food, the body turns to its protein stores to provide energy and you start to "eat" your own muscles.

4 Certain exercises burn fat from specific areas

The theory behind "spot reducing" is that muscle activity in a specific area stimulates the burning of the fat deposits closest to that muscle. So, to slim down your thighs, you cycle, or to flatten your stomach, you do sit-ups. Sadly, the body does not work like this. You cannot choose where you would like the fat to come from when you work out. Exercise stimulates a general rather than a specific use of fat, through hormones delivered in the bloodstream to the whole body. Exercise will, however, build lean tissue, which influences the metabolic rate (see Myth 8, opposite). Strengthening certain areas, such as the abdominals and the hamstrings, also improves posture and this in itself will have a positive effect on your appearance.

5 Some diets target weight from one body area, e.g. the hips

This idea could be part of Myth 4. Unfortunately, the theory doesn't add up and it is about as possible as emptying one side of a bottle.

6 Grapefruit and egg (substitute any food) is a magic combination for weight loss

"One-food-centred" diets are based on the idea that particular foods, or combinations of them, magically burn off fat. The theory is that the process of digesting certain foods requires more calories than they contain. You can lose weight fast on diets like these: they are very-low-calorie diets that border dangerously on starvation and you won't lose the weight permanently. Apart from being repetitious and boring, these diets seriously lack nutrients, slow down your metabolism and provide very little energy.

7 The body cannot digest certain foods at the same time

This "food combining" theory is based on the idea that the digestive enzymes that break down protein and carbohydrates neutralize each other, leaving undigested foods to ferment in the gut, become toxic and cause obesity and constipation. Medical opinion states that this type of diet only works because it makes the dieter monitor the quality and quantity of food they eat.

8 My metabolism is so slow I can't lose weight

Everyone claims to have a friend who "eats like a horse and never gains weight", but scientists are still looking for this person. Depending on age and gender, we all burn food at about the same rate. This is because our metabolic rate is linked to our lean tissue; women naturally have less muscle and more fat than men, and muscle tends to decrease with age. Muscle burns fuel faster than fat does because it is a working part of the body – fat is just something we carry around. Dramatic weight loss through dieting depletes muscle mass, lowering the metabolic rate. The body learns to survive on fewer calories and, after the diet, healthy amounts of food become surplus to requirements and are stored as fat. You regain weight quickly.

9 Wearing plastic or sweat gear helps weight loss

Forcing yourself to sweat makes you lose water, not fat. Water is essential to life and you can drink as much as you like – it contains no calories and no fat.

10 Exercise is a useless way to lose weight: you have to burn 3,500 calories to lose just 0.45kg/1lb of fat

It is true that 0.45kg (1lb) of fat is worth about 3,500 calories. If you are used to starvation diets, where the scales show a loss of five times this amount in a week, you might be disheartened. The only way you can lose that much "weight" in a week, however, is by losing muscle and water, and all the evidence shows it will very quickly return. Combining exercise with dieting means more of the weight lost will be fat. Remember, the scales don't tell the whole truth: muscle is heavier than fat. 0.45 kg (1lb) of fat takes up 508 cubic cm (31 cubic inches) of space – about the size of a cabbage. 0.45kg (1lb) of muscle only takes up 410 cubic cm (25 cubic inches). So, if you replaced 2.25kg (5lb) of fat with 2.25kg (5lb) of muscle, you would weigh the same but you would be around 492 cubic cm (30 cubic inches) smaller. Think about it.

The Facts

There is no secret formula for weight loss. You cannot lose weight without creating a "calorie deficit" – burning off more calories than you take in as food. In theory, you can choose one of three ways to do this: eat less, exercise more, or combine the two by eating a little less while exercising a little more. When the facts are laid out, the choice is obvious.

In contrast to all the myths about weight loss, there is one central fact:

Combining a reduced intake of food, that is high in carbohydrates and low in fat, with an appropriate exercise programme is the only way to lose body fat and lose it permanently.

A diet high in carbohydrates will give you plenty of energy to exercise. The benefits of exercise are twofold: it burns fat as a fuel and at the same time maintains muscle mass, so that your metabolic rate remains high, despite the fact that you are losing weight. It may not be as seductive as all those lose weight fast diets but it really is the closest you will ever get to a magic formula for permanent weight loss.

The practical method

No doctor would recommend that you lose more than about ½ – 1kg (about 1 – 2lb) of weight per week. 0.45kg (1lb) of fat represents approximately 3,500 calories. This may seem a vast amount of calories but, spread over a week, it averages out at no more than 500 calories per day. By combining the right type of exercise with the right type of diet, you can achieve this quite easily without either starving yourself or killing yourself in the gym.

It might seem like a slow process but you cannot lose weight quickly and lose it permanently. If you lose fat rather than muscle and water, you can be sure that the weight will stay off. Bear in mind that 0.45kg (1lb) of fat is equal to 508 cubic cm (31 cubic inches) of body mass, so over 10 weeks you could lose a massive 5,080 cubic cm (310 cubic inches) of fat. Now that is a lot of fat.

If you want to lose 0.45kg (1lb) of fat in a week, your calorie deficit should be 500 calories per day. You can achieve this by doing the following:

■ Decrease the energy you take in by 250 calories a day. Stick to foods that are high in carbohydrates and low in fat (see pages 38 – 39). Fat has over twice the calories of carbohydrates, so cutting down on fat is the simplest and healthiest way to reduce calories. Some carbohydrates release energy gradually, which keeps your blood-sugar level constant so you will not suffer from the sugar cravings, hunger and weakness that plague most attempts to lose weight.

■ At the same time, increase the energy you use every day by 250 calories. This is easily done with 30 minutes of moderate aerobic exercise, such as cycling or jogging, or with an hour's brisk walk. However unfit you feel, you can embark on an exercise programme that will build up safely to achieve this (see page 55).

The benefits of losing weight in this way are numerous:

High energy A diet high in carbohydrates gives you maximum energy. In contrast, a low-calorie diet delivers exactly what it promises: low energy. A diet that makes you weak and hungry leaves you open to temptation, and usually results in bingeing, when the body's survival instinct takes over and does its best to persuade you to eat.

Weight loss is permanent A diet high in carbohydrates provides plenty of energy to exercise, which helps to ensure that weight stays off. Quick-fix diets usually mean that you regain weight just as quickly as you lost it.

Body fat is substantially decreased You can be sure that you are losing fat. Shorter periods of calorie restriction alone have been shown to result in temporary weight loss, mainly from muscle and water.

Exercise re-educates the body If you exercise, your natural appetite cues are reprogrammed to respond to the need for food, while the appetite of an inactive person tends to "freewheel". A programme of weight loss that includes exercise relies less on reducing calories, so there is less hunger and less temptation.

Muscle mass is maintained Aerobic exercise preserves muscle mass, while fat is burnt as a fuel, so your metabolic rate remains high.

Significant health benefits Unique benefits are achieved by increasing exercise and reducing fat. These include a reduced risk of several obesity-linked diseases that can endanger the heart. Weight-bearing exercise also maintains bone mass and helps guard against osteoporosis in old age.

Exercise releases endorphins These "feel-good" hormones give you an increased sense of wellbeing. Exercise also provides an outlet from the stresses of everyday life and a good work out will leave you feeling physically and mentally refreshed. You will also benefit from the positive feeling of actively contributing to your weight loss.

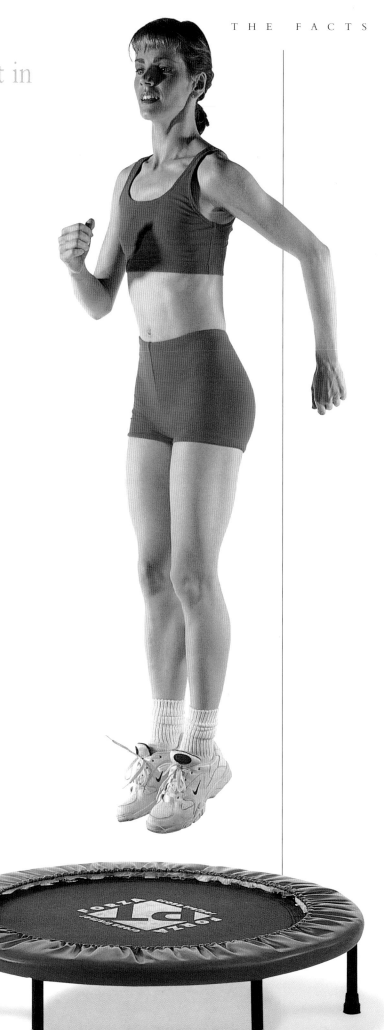

Using Energy

Muscles make up almost half of the body mass. There are over 660 different muscles in the human body and, even at rest, they account for about 20% of the average daily energy you use. During intense exercise, this can increase one hundredfold. The more exercise you do, the more energy the muscles burn.

Fuel for life

Although energy is usually associated with exercise, it is also used when you are at rest. Just as a car burns fuel even when the engine is idling, the body uses energy even when you are asleep, simply in order to stay alive. This energy is not conjured up from thin air: it comes from your daily diet. The food you eat goes through a digestive process in which the useful parts are extracted and the waste expelled. Anything beyond what you need gets stored for future use.

Storing energy

Muscles are made up of 75% protein and 20% water. They are dense and compact: 0.45kg (1lb) of muscle is 98 cubic cm (6 cubic inches) smaller in volume than 0.45kg (1lb) of fat. In the short term, a limited amount of carbohydrates can be stored in the muscles. The only long-term storage system the body has is fat. Its capacity to store fat is practically unlimited and it is the ultimate destination of any food that is surplus to requirements. The average person has 2,000 calories' worth of carbohydrates stored, compared to about 80,000 calories' worth of fat. That's enough carbohydrates to run 20 miles, and more than enough fat to run the length of Great Britain.

Burning fat: the problem

It may seem hard to believe, but the body actually prefers to use fat for energy. It likes to save the carbohydrates to feed the brain, which needs around 120g (4oz) daily – the sugar in ten apples. We worry, quite rightly, when the brain is starved of oxygen, yet people often go on diets that starve the brain of sugar.

The body has vast stores of fat available and wants to use them, so why is obesity such a problem? Firstly, it is because technology has eliminated most of the fat-burning activities from modern life; we can have clean clothes at the touch of a button and rarely walk anywhere. We're left with time on our hands and, as a direct consequence, flab on our hips. At the same time, food is cheaper and more plentiful than ever and we eat rich and fatty foods every day. We are simply eating more fat than we burn. The result is an alarming increase in obesity that is beginning to rival even smoking-related diseases as a cause of death.

The solution

The one method of weight control that is proven to be successful in the long term, works because it doesn't try to ignore the laws of nature. By combining a high-carbohydrate, low-fat diet with the right type of exercise, you can tackle both the major causes of obesity, so weight loss will be permanent. You can ignore all the "miracle" cures: when the facts are set out, you will find that they are too persuasive to ignore.

The Muscle Groups

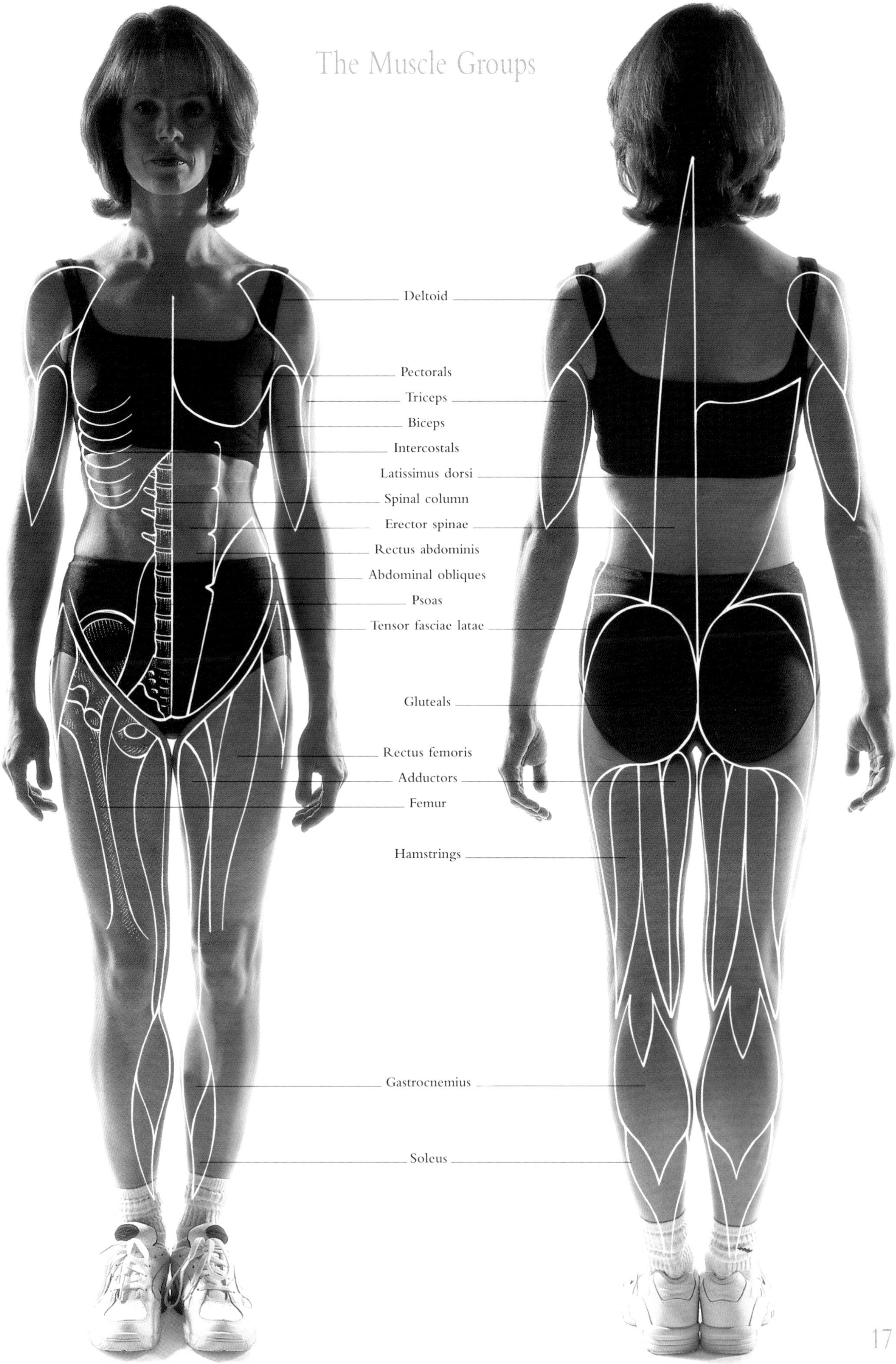

Deltoid

Pectorals

Triceps

Biceps

Intercostals

Latissimus dorsi

Spinal column

Erector spinae

Rectus abdominis

Abdominal obliques

Psoas

Tensor fasciae latae

Gluteals

Rectus femoris

Adductors

Femur

Hamstrings

Gastrocnemius

Soleus

Reading Your Heart Rate

If you want to lose body fat permanently, you have to use it as a fuel in aerobic endurance exercise (see page 21). Your watch tells you how long you are working – the endurance element – and it can also help you check that you aren't working too hard.

Hitting the right intensity

You find out how hard you are working by measuring your heart rate. During exercise, your heart rate goes up; the harder you work, the faster the heart beats. Everyone has a maximum heart rate – the fastest it can possibly beat. Calculating how close your heart rate is to its maximum during exercise enables you to check the intensity of your work out.

Reading your heart rate

Your training heart rate must be measured during exercise, but you may find it useful to take a few practice readings while resting. It takes time to become proficient and initial attempts may be a little far-fetched.

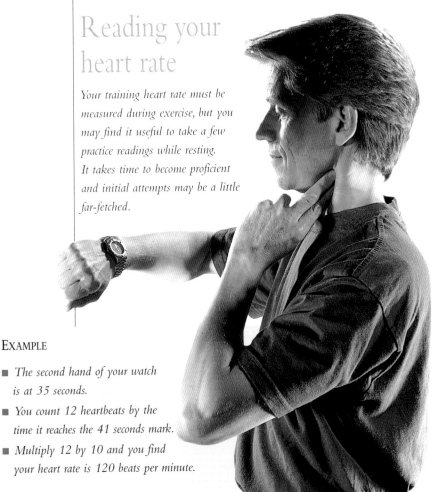

1 *Find your pulse either on the underside of your wrist, or on the side of your neck. Use your first two fingers, not the thumb, as it has its own pulse which can distort the accuracy of a reading. You may need to make a brief stop, but take your pulse immediately.*

2 *Start counting your pulse when the second hand of your watch reaches a given point, and count the beats over the next six seconds.*

3 *Multiply this number by 10 to work out the number of beats in 60 seconds and you have the beats per minute (BPM). This is your heart rate. You can test the accuracy by counting the beats over 30 seconds and multiplying them by 2 to see if you get the same result.*

EXAMPLE

- *The second hand of your watch is at 35 seconds.*
- *You count 12 heartbeats by the time it reaches the 41 seconds mark.*
- *Multiply 12 by 10 and you find your heart rate is 120 beats per minute.*

Using a heart-rate monitor

You can also check your heart rate using an electronic heart-rate monitor. This will give an accurate read-out of your heart rate throughout exercise. Different models are available but you only need the most basic (and the cheapest).

1 *Strap the transmitter band of the monitor around your chest, directly next to your skin. This will relay information to the monitor.*

2 *Strap the monitor, which resembles a digital watch, to your wrist. The display will show you a constant reading of your heart rate.*

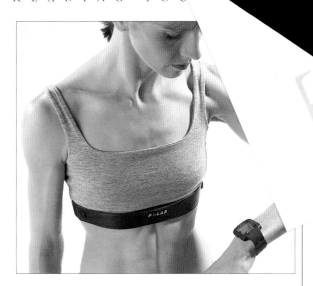

Your maximum heart rate

To calculate if you are working at the right intensity, you also need to know your maximum heart rate. Although there are tests to measure this, they aren't necessary unless you have a heart problem; instead, it can be estimated. As you get older, the maximum rate at which your heart can beat decreases, so the age-based formula on the right works as a guideline.

Your age-predicted maximum heart rate = (220 - your age)

- *If you are 18 years old, your age-predicted maximum will be:* **220 - 18 = 202 BPM**
- *If you are 25 years old:* **220 - 25 = 195 BPM**
- *If you are 35 years old:* **220 - 35 = 185 BPM**
- *If you are 50 years old:* **220 - 50 = 170 BPM**
- *If you are 65 years old:* **220 - 65 = 155 BPM**

Target zones for different types of exercise

In anaerobic exercise

Your heart is working faster than 85% of its maximum heart rate (see above):

Running up the stairs

Sprinting

Push-starting the car

- *If you are 18 years old:* at least **171 BPM**
- *If you are 25 years old:* at least **165 BPM**
- *If you are 35 years old:* at least **157 BPM**
- *If you are 50 years old:* at least **144 BPM**
- *If you are 65 years old:* at least **131 BPM**

In aerobic exercise

Your heart is working between 60% and 85% of its maximum heart rate (see above):

Walking the dog

Jogging

Cycling to the shops

- *If you are 18 years old:* between **121 and 171 BPM**
- *If you are 25 years old:* between **117 and 165 BPM**
- *If you are 35 years old:* between **111 and 157 BPM**
- *If you are 50 years old:* between **102 and 144 BPM**
- *If you are 65 years old:* between **93 and 131 BPM**

In aerobic endurance exercise

Your heart is working between 60% and 70% of its maximum heart rate (see above) for at least 20 minutes:

An hour's walk

30 minutes of cycling

A country hike

- *If you are 18 years old:* between **121 and 141 BPM**
- *If you are 25 years old:* between **117 and 136 BPM**
- *If you are 35 years old:* between **111 and 129 BPM**
- *If you are 50 years old:* between **102 and 119 BPM**
- *If you are 65 years old:* between **93 and 108 BPM**

CAUTION

If you have a family history of heart problems, check with your GP before starting any exercise programme.

Energy for Life

Total Nutrition Guide

Most of us have, at some time in our lives, suffered the hunger pangs that come with a "low-calorie diet" yet, despite all the effort it involves, dieting is usually a short-term solution to a long-term problem. Sustained, healthy weight control lies in finding the right balance between the different types of food you eat.

But how can you translate this theory to the food on your plate? Traditional diets rely on obsessively counting calories, yet there is a much simpler way. Understanding the essentials of healthy eating was, for me, the key to controlling my weight without losing energy, and I haven't felt hungry since.

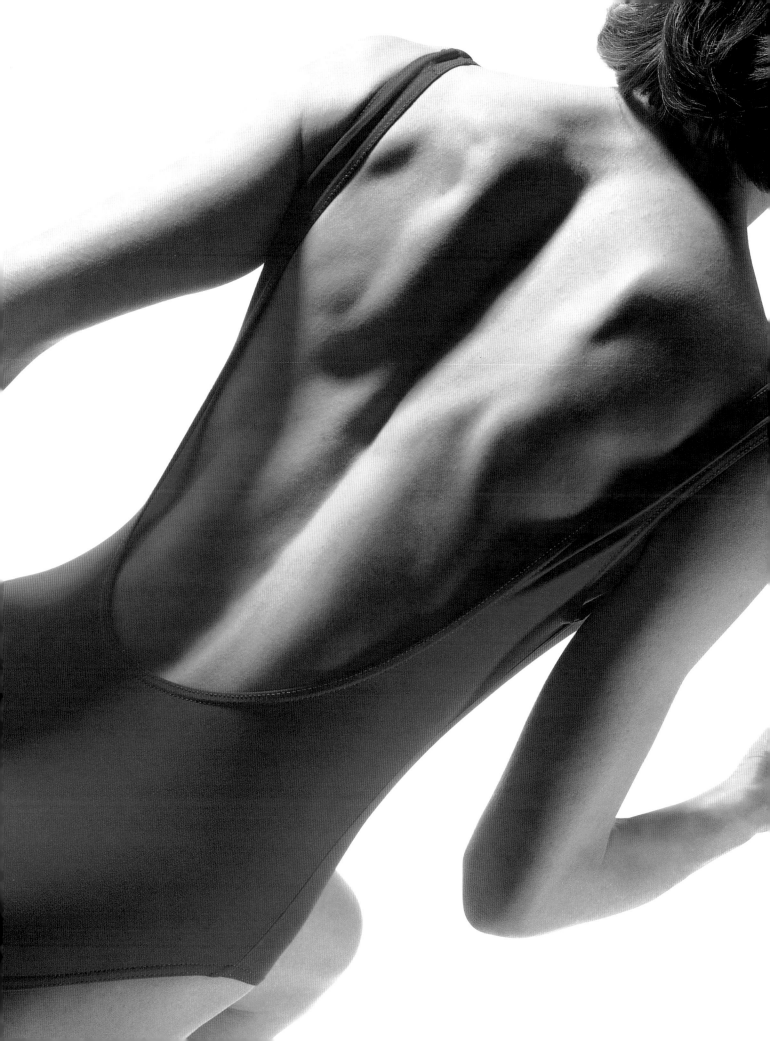

The Low-down on Calories

For most people, "going on a diet" means counting and cutting calories. Filled with optimism and determination, they clear the fridge of anything vaguely appetizing and load it up with foods that boast they "help slimming as part of a calorie-controlled diet".

What is a calorie?

You can certainly lose weight on a calorie-controlled diet, although for how long is open to question. Unfortunately, you'll also lose the most important thing that calories supply: energy. Despite years of obsessively counting them, most dieters are still not very clear on exactly what a calorie is. Before you decide to cut them, it might be a good idea to find out.

Cutting energy

Most of the food you buy (and certainly all the packaged food) tells you how many calories it contains. You'll find it listed under one of three words: "kcals", "kjoules" or "energy". The last of these provides the clue. The calorific content of food doesn't indicate how fat you'll get if you eat that food; it tells you how much energy it will provide. This is why cutting calories inevitably means cutting energy; the two words are interchangeable. In nutritional terms, calories measure the energy provided by the food you eat to "heat" or fuel your body. "Calorific expenditure" is the amount of energy you use.

If that was the end of the story, you could argue that the more calories you eat, the more energy you have and, in a way, you would be right. You would certainly have a lot of potential energy, but recent research shows that you would be unlikely to use it. We burn far fewer calories every week than our grandparents did, and our lifestyles rarely include the sort of long-term activity that burns fat. Most of the energy we use comes from carbohydrates. Unfortunately, less useful calories don't just disappear. You either use them or you store them, and the only long-term storage system we have is body fat.

Where do calories come from?

With one exception, calories come from three sources: carbohydrates, protein and fat provide all the energy, and therefore the calories, your body needs, but the recipe for good health has three other essential ingredients: vitamins, minerals and water. The absence of any one of these six elements would eventually lead to illness and, in the long term, would prove fatal. Vitamins, minerals and water play an important part in just about everything that goes on in the body but, contrary to popular belief, they do not supply energy; they are calorie-free, and energy comes only with calories.

Alcohol also supplies a considerable number of calories but it contributes very little to sound nutrition. If you're trying to lose weight, you should try to drink as little alcohol as possible.

Although most food can be categorized as predominantly carbohydrates, protein or fat, there are very few that are made up of only one of these. In most cases, the calories come from two or three sources. To control your weight, it's not the number of calories you should be watching, but where they come from. Some calories are just more useful than others.

How many calories do you need?

Your body uses energy simply to stay alive. The resting metabolic rate tells you how many calories your body would use if you spent the entire day lying down. To get an idea of how much energy you really use, you have to add on the energy required in day-to-day living – getting up and going to work, for instance – and the energy you use in eating and digesting food. These three elements make up your total daily energy expenditure.

Survival tactics

It is highly unlikely that, as an adult, your body can maintain itself on fewer than 1,200 calories a day. If you try to survive on less than this, you will be hard-pushed to get all the nutrients you require for long-term health. In addition, taking in fewer calories than your body needs encourages it to break down protein (your muscles) to supply energy. As they influence your metabolism, depleting the muscles leads to a lowering of your metabolic rate.

Dramatic weight loss through diet alone has been proven to have a serious and sustained effect on the metabolism, above and beyond the effect of losing lean tissue. The body is designed to survive famine, even if it is self-inflicted. In severe diets, the metabolic rate can be depressed by as much as 45% as the body becomes more "energy efficient", slowing down its systems to enable it to survive on fewer calories. It's a bit like driving a car which is low on petrol. If you want to make it last until the nearest garage, you have no option but to drive very slowly. The lower the speed, the less fuel you burn. As your metabolic rate goes down, the body uses less energy, and you will find it harder to lose weight, however little you eat. Regular exercise, on the other hand, can raise your metabolic rate by maintaining, and even increasing, muscle mass.

ESTIMATING YOUR RESTING METABOLIC RATE (RMR)

You can estimate your RMR by multiplying your weight in pounds by 10 (1lb = 0.45kg)

- *If you weigh 130lb, your RMR will be approximately 1,300 calories: 130 X 10 = 1,300*

Remember, the resting metabolic rate is not your ideal calorie intake; it only tells you how many calories you would use to lie in bed all day.

How the body uses energy

Between 60 – 75 % of the energy you use in a day is taken up in staying alive. Physical activity – working, shopping or exercising – accounts for a further 15 – 30%, depending on how active you are, and a small amount of energy is used to digest food. By far the easiest way to increase your energy expenditure is to add on exercise; builders and endurance athletes can use twice as much energy every day as the average adult.

RESTING METABOLIC RATE USES 60 – 75% OF TOTAL DAILY ENERGY

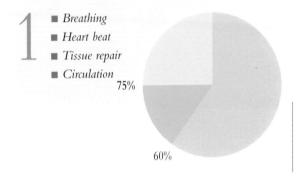

1
- Breathing
- Heart beat
- Tissue repair
- Circulation

75%

60%

PHYSICAL ACTIVITY USES 15 – 30% OF TOTAL DAILY ENERGY

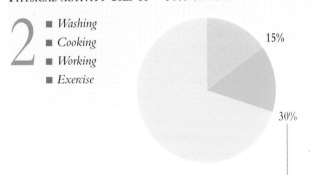

2
- Washing
- Cooking
- Working
- Exercise

15%

30%

EATING AND DIGESTING FOOD USES 10% OF TOTAL DAILY ENERGY

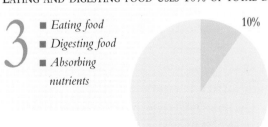

3
- Eating food
- Digesting food
- Absorbing nutrients

10%

Carbohydrates

This is a catch-all term for starchy and sweet foods, from pasta to sugar lumps. Carbohydrates are the major fuel for all physical activity – not just the kind of exercise that athletes do, but running for the bus as well. A low-carbohydrate diet leads to low energy, which leads to low activity – this is how weight creeps up.

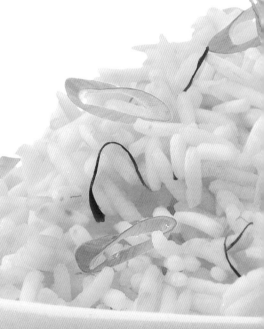

What do they do?

■ Stored in the liver and muscles as glycogen, carbohydrates serve as a major energy source for all activity.

■ Carbohydrates are the main fuel of the central nervous system, which includes the brain.

■ They are an essential part of the fat-burning process and serve as a "primer": if carbohydrates are not present, fat cannot be broken down completely.

■ They provide 4 calories of energy per gram.

Where are they found?

Nature has given us three types of carbohydrates, all of which can be called "unrefined".

"Simple" carbohydrates

Often referred to collectively as "simple sugars", these include: glucose (a sugar that occurs naturally in foods such as fruit), fructose (another natural sugar in fruit), lactose (present in milk, including breast milk) and sucrose (found in sugar cane).

"Complex" carbohydrates

These are also known as starches. Plants store carbohydrates as starch, and it is found in rice, flour and potatoes. Starch is made up of a chain of simple sugars that are linked together, so it is slower to break down and releases its energy over a longer period.

Dietary fibre

An integral part of most unrefined carbohydrates, fibre is found in the cell walls of vegetables, fruit, beans and wholegrain cereals. Most fibre cannot be digested by humans but it is still extremely beneficial. It provides bulk that makes you feel full and naturally limits the amount you eat at any one time. Fibre also acts as a binding agent and speeds up the passage of food through the intestines. In this way, fibre helps to guard against gastrointestinal disease and colon cancer.

Refined sugar

Man has managed to introduce a fourth carbohydrate into the diet. Refined sugar, such as table sugar, is not found in nature, which is a good indication of just how much your body needs it. It is used to add sweetness to confectionery, cakes, biscuits and a good deal of supposedly savoury food. It provides plenty of calories and therefore plenty of energy, but contributes no nutritional value to your diet, as refined carbohydrates are stripped of all their vitamins, minerals and fibre. Refined sugar releases its energy very quickly, triggering an abrupt insulin response that can lead to light-headedness and "blood sugar jitters" (see page 54). After an initial high, your energy levels will feel lower than they did before you ate, until they eventually stabilize.

Unrefined vs refined carbohydrates

Unrefined carbohydrates, such as wholemeal bread, wholewheat pasta, wholegrain cereals, brown rice and fruit, provide valuable vitamins and minerals along with energy. The process of refining wholewheat flour into white flour, for example, strips it of nutrients, leaving little else apart from calories. This is one of the reasons why unrefined carbohydrates are a much healthier choice.

Weight control

As well as providing vitamins and minerals, unrefined carbohydrates contribute fibre to the diet, which is an important factor in appetite control (and in curbing weight gain). I find it impossible to overeat on unrefined carbohydrates – they are almost self-limiting. You feel full much sooner after a meal of unrefined carbohydrates than after one based on protein, fat or refined sugar, so you can satisfy your appetite without overloading on calories. A jacket potato, for example, has the same amount of energy/calories as an iced doughnut but, whereas a doughnut is mainly sugar and fat, a potato is high in fibre and complex carbohydrates. You might be able to eat two or three doughnuts, but you would be hard-pushed to manage more than one large baked potato. Foods high in unrefined carbohydrates are not only more filling, they are also usually lower in fat.

CARBOHYDRATE
FOODS TO LIMIT IN
YOUR DIET

■

SUGAR
(WHITE & BROWN)

■

SWEETS

■

CHOCOLATE

■

CAKES

■

SWEET BISCUITS

■

SUGARY DRINKS

■

JAM

■

HONEY

■

SYRUPS

Protein

The role of protein – maintaining and repairing tissue – cannot be fulfilled by any other nutrient, but there is no benefit at all from eating excessive amounts. Protein won't give you more energy or stronger muscles and it can be detrimental rather than beneficial to health.

In fact, you need much less protein than you may imagine.

What does it do?

■ Protein maintains, repairs and builds the living tissue in the body but, contrary to popular opinion, you don't increase muscle bulk by eating extra protein.
■ It is the main component of muscles, tendons and ligaments.
■ Protein can be converted to glucose and can provide energy for both the muscles and the brain when you eat insufficient amounts of carbohydrates. The use of protein for energy will take precedence over its foremost task of maintaining tissues, which means injuries and wounds will be slow to heal.
■ Protein provides 4 calories of energy per gram.

Where is it found?

Protein is present in most foods. It is made up of several amino acids, the building blocks of living tissue. You need around 20 different amino acids and they can be split into two categories. Eight of them (nine for children) cannot be made within the body, so you have to get them from what you eat. They are known as "essential" amino acids. This does not mean that the remaining twelve are not necessary – they are all vital for health, but the others can be manufactured in the body from the essential amino acids in your diet.

Protein quality

Foods contain amino acids in varying proportions and the quality of a protein is measured by how closely the amino acids match the human body's requirements. The closer the match, the more efficiently it can be used. The amino acids in animal proteins, such as eggs, milk, cheese, meat, poultry and fish, are very similar to human requirements. They are said to have a high "biological value", and may be described as "complete" proteins. Protein from plant sources is not generally as well-matched but, as meals are usually based around a variety of foods

---

LOW-FAT SOURCES OF PROTEIN

Remove the fat or skin from meat and poultry, and use a low-fat method of cooking, such as steaming or grilling, to prepare food.

■

VERY LEAN MEAT

■

FISH

■

SKINLESS POULTRY

■

TOFU

■

PEAS & BEANS

■

LOW-FAT DAIRY PRODUCTS

■

SMALL AMOUNTS OF PROTEIN ARE ALSO FOUND IN BREAD, PASTA & BREAKFAST CEREALS

DAILY REQUIREMENT

Protein should make up 10 – 20% of the daily diet.

such as bread with cheese, rice with lentils, or vegetables with pasta, it is not difficult to get a well-balanced mix of amino acids, even if you don't eat meat. You don't need to balance the amino acids in every meal, but the greater the variety of protein sources in your diet, the better.

The best sources of protein

Protein is present, to some degree, in almost everything you eat; the only foods that contain absolutely no protein are vegetable and nut oils, and refined table sugar. Protein is not particularly high in most fruit and vegetables, although foods from other plant sources, such as beans, wholegrain cereals, rice and pasta, contain a significant amount of it. Vegetarians and vegans who eat a wide variety of these foods should not be protein-deficient, especially if they eat soya beans, which are as high in protein as eggs and cheese.

The great protein myth

Despite the wealth of sensible information that is available, there is a persistent misunderstanding about protein and how much is really needed: ideally, it should only make up between 10 – 20% of what you eat.

Since the heyday of the high-protein/low-carbohydrate diet in the Seventies, grilled steak and lean chicken have been the cornerstone of the slimmer's diet. Potatoes and pasta continue to be seen as no-go areas for anyone watching their weight yet, while many high-carbohydrate foods contain only a trace of fat, high-protein foods are often a source of hidden fat. Even lean beef derives about 50% of its calories from fat, and the other 50% from protein. Although protein is certainly an important part of the diet – we couldn't function without it – according to recent US research, when the most popular types of diet were compared, the high-protein/low-carbohydrate diet was the only one for which no advantages could be found.

In a high-protein regime, when you restrict the amount of carbohydrates you eat, the body is forced to use protein as an energy source. The stores of carbohydrates (about 2,000 calories' worth) are used up in about 24 hours. The brain needs a constant level of sugar in the blood and, when it isn't provided in the diet, the body supplies it by converting protein into glucose. This diverts protein from its main task of repairing and maintaining tissue. In extreme cases of starvation, the body turns to its protein stores, the muscles, to provide energy. Losing muscle mass through dieting can lead to a lowering of the metabolic rate and can be dangerous.

Weight control

Today, 70% of the protein we eat is derived from animal produce; seventy years ago, it came equally from plants and animals. As meat products contain not only protein but also fat, many of us are eating much higher levels of saturated fat than we need. It is hardly surprising that up to a quarter of adults in the Western world are considered overweight and that heart disease is now a major cause of death in most industrialized nations.

HIGH-FAT SOURCES
OF PROTEIN

FATTY MEAT

EGGS

FULL-FAT DAIRY
PRODUCTS

NUTS

Fat

As much as everyone loves to hate it, fat is suprisingly palatable; it adds flavour and texture to the food we eat. A little fat is vital for good health, but as fat is present in most foods, especially those high in protein, it creeps into your diet more than you realize. Unless you eat a very limited diet, you should get enough fat without trying.

What does it do?

- Certain fatty acids are essential: they cannot be made in the body yet are needed to help form cell walls and for growth, sexual reproduction and skin maintenance.
- The fat-soluble vitamins A, D, E and K are carried in fat.
- Fat is important as a fuel in light and moderate long-term activity.
- At 9 calories per gram, fat provides over twice as much energy as carbohydrates.

Where is it found?

There are two types of fat: saturated and unsaturated. Unsaturated fat is no lower in calories than any other fat, but it's a better choice, as saturated fat can raise blood cholesterol levels which can lead to heart disease. For good health, at least two-thirds of the fat you eat should be unsaturated.

Saturated fat

Found mainly in animal and dairy products, like butter, lard, cheese, fatty meat, eggs and whole milk, saturated fat tends to be solid at room temperature: the firmer the fat, the more saturated it is. There are some exceptions to this – palm and coconut oil are high in saturated fat, despite being liquid.

Unsaturated fat

There are two types of unsaturated fat: polyunsaturated and monounsaturated, and they are usually liquid at room temperature. Olive oil is probably the best-known source of monounsaturated fat; other sources include rapeseed oil and sesame oil. Polyunsaturated fat includes sunflower oil, soya oil, safflower oil, corn oil, walnut oil, peanut oil and fish oil. Replacing saturated with unsaturated fat can reduce the level of LDL, or "bad", cholesterol, the type that leads to narrowing of the arteries. The omega-3 fatty acids found in cold-water fish, such as tuna, herring, mackerel and sardines, are thought to have a beneficial effect on health, lowering the risk of heart disease.

SOURCES OF UNSATURATED FAT

- VEGETABLE OILS
- OLIVE OIL
- NUT OILS
- AVOCADO
- NUTS
- SEEDS
- OILY FISH, SUCH AS TUNA, HERRING MACKEREL & SARDINES

DAILY REQUIREMENT

Fat should make up no more than 30% of your diet. If you are trying to lose weight, you may want to eat even less.

Hydrogenated fat

Most margarines and spreads contain a mixture of fats, yet advertize that they are "high in polyunsaturates". The process of hydrogenation makes liquid fats solid enough to be sold in a tub rather than a bottle. It adds hydrogen, which converts unsaturated fat into saturated fat, making it less beneficial to health. Hydrogenated fat is also found in foods such as sausages, pies, biscuits and cakes.

Cholesterol

A vital substance in the body, cholesterol is made by all animals, including humans. If your diet is high in saturated fat, the liver is stimulated to make more cholesterol than the body needs. The level of cholesterol in the blood goes up, and cholesterol-rich deposits are formed in the arteries which supply the heart with blood. This causes them to narrow, and can eventually lead to a heart attack. Saturated fat has a more harmful effect than the cholesterol found in foods, but substituting unsaturated fats can help to lower blood cholesterol levels. Cholesterol is not found in plant foods.

Lowering your fat intake

There are two major reasons why you should keep the fat you eat to a minimum: it is bad for your health, and it leads to weight gain. Any excess food you eat will be stored as body fat, however, fat is more easily converted to body fat than any other nutrient. The best way to lose weight is to replace fat with carbohydrate-rich foods and many foods are now available in reduced or low-fat versions. Some stores highlight items that are naturally low in fat but, beware, when fat is removed or reduced, it is often (not always) replaced with refined sugar. The list below gives alternatives that are no less filling, but that are much less fattening:

SOURCES OF SATURATED FAT

- FATTY CUTS OF MEAT
- MEAT PRODUCTS, SUCH AS SAUSAGES & PIES
- FULL-FAT DAIRY PRODUCTS
- BUTTER
- SOME MARGARINES
- PALM OIL
- COCONUT OIL
- BISCUITS
- CAKES
- SAVOURY SNACKS

CUT OUT	REPLACE WITH
Croissants	Low-fat bagels
Butter or margarine	Low-fat spread
Full-fat dairy products	Low-fat dairy products
Cream- or oil-based salad dressings	Yoghurt-based or low-fat dressings
Chips	Potatoes, boiled or baked
Cheese or cream sauces	Vegetable-based sauces
Fried fish or meat	Grilled fish or meat
Fatty meat, sausages or pies	Poultry without skin, lean cuts of meat
Sweets, snacks and crisps	Fruit, rice cakes, vegetables

Vitamins & Minerals An essential

part of every process that happens in the body, these nutrients are vital for

good health. Supplements are rarely

necessary, as a varied diet normally

provides all you need.

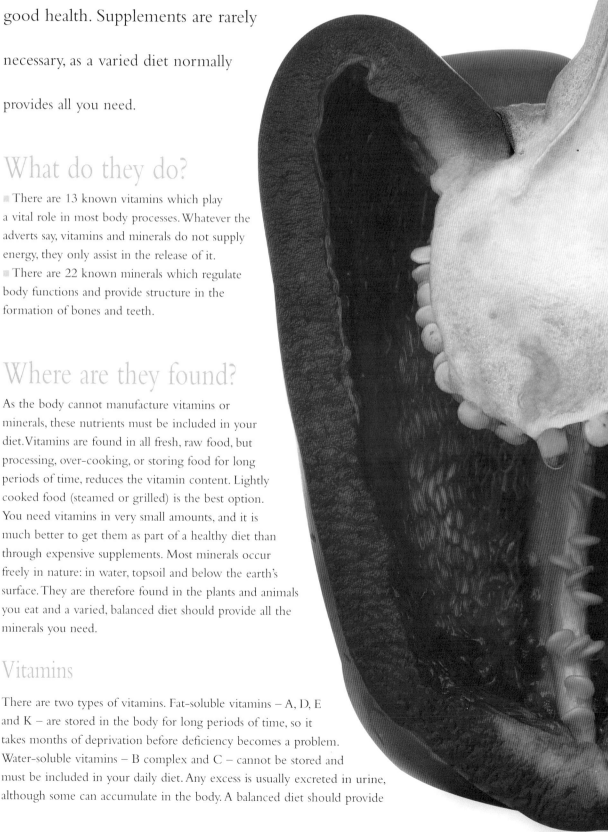

GOOD SOURCES OF VITAMINS & MINERALS

■
RAW FRUIT & VEGETABLES

■
LIGHTLY COOKED, FRESH OR FROZEN FRUIT & VEGETABLES

■
WHOLEGRAIN CEREALS & GRAINS

■
LOW-FAT DAIRY PRODUCTS

■
BEANS & PEAS

■
LEAN MEAT

What do they do?

■ There are 13 known vitamins which play a vital role in most body processes. Whatever the adverts say, vitamins and minerals do not supply energy, they only assist in the release of it.
■ There are 22 known minerals which regulate body functions and provide structure in the formation of bones and teeth.

Where are they found?

As the body cannot manufacture vitamins or minerals, these nutrients must be included in your diet. Vitamins are found in all fresh, raw food, but processing, over-cooking, or storing food for long periods of time, reduces the vitamin content. Lightly cooked food (steamed or grilled) is the best option. You need vitamins in very small amounts, and it is much better to get them as part of a healthy diet than through expensive supplements. Most minerals occur freely in nature: in water, topsoil and below the earth's surface. They are therefore found in the plants and animals you eat and a varied, balanced diet should provide all the minerals you need.

DAILY REQUIREMENT
Eat five or more different fruit and vegetables each day to ensure a good intake of vitamins and minerals. Choose fresh or frozen in preference to canned (see pages 38 – 39).

Vitamins

There are two types of vitamins. Fat-soluble vitamins – A, D, E and K – are stored in the body for long periods of time, so it takes months of deprivation before deficiency becomes a problem. Water-soluble vitamins – B complex and C – cannot be stored and must be included in your daily diet. Any excess is usually excreted in urine, although some can accumulate in the body. A balanced diet should provide all the vitamins you need. If you think you need a supplement, limit yourself to a multi-vitamin that provides the recommended daily amount. Diagnosing individual vitamin deficiencies is best left to your doctor, as overdoses can be toxic.

Minerals

A balanced diet should provide you with sufficient minerals, but you should pay particular attention to your intake of calcium and iron.

Calcium

Vital for nerve transmission and blood clotting, calcium also gives bones their strength. If you do not eat sufficient calcium, the body steals it from the bones. This can lead to osteoporosis, a condition that makes the bones fragile and prone to fracture. Osteoporosis does affect men, however, women are at greater risk, especially if they are very thin, eat insufficient calcium-rich foods, drink too much caffeine, or smoke. The female hormone oestrogen, which has a protective effect on bone-mass, is reduced after the menopause. Women who do not menstruate regularly are also particularly vulnerable and should consult a doctor. The best defence against osteoporosis is to combine a good calcium intake with weight-bearing exercise, such as brisk walking, which stimulates bone formation. Women should try to maximize bone strength during their twenties.

Sources: Milk, dairy produce (low-fat versions contain just as much), sardines and canned salmon (as long as you eat the bones), tofu, green leafy vegetables and beans. You need about 800mg of calcium a day.

Iron

As this mineral is lost during menstruation, iron deficiency is fairly common in women. This is one of the few instances when a doctor may prescribe a supplement.

Sources: Red meat, liver, egg yolk, green leafy vegetables, bread, beans, fortified breakfast cereal and some dried fruit. The iron in non-meat produce is not as well-absorbed by the body, but you can increase its absorption by eating or drinking a source of vitamin C, such as a glass of orange juice, at the same time. A simple way to increase iron intake is to cook with unenamelled, cast-iron saucepans.

Salt

Sweating causes the body to lose salt, but the need for added salt is probably more imagined than real. Most of us eat twice as much salt as we need. Excess sodium (a component of salt) can lead to high blood pressure, which in turn can increase the risk of strokes.

Sources: Watch out for added salt in smoked fish, savoury snacks and in many processed foods.

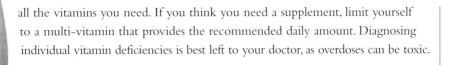

FOODS WITH A
REDUCED VITAMIN &
MINERAL CONTENT

▪

FOOD STORED FOR
A LONG TIME

▪

OVER-COOKED FOOD

▪

FOOD KEPT WARM
FOR A LONG TIME

▪

CANNED FOOD

▪

PROCESSED FOOD

▪

PEELED FRUIT
& VEGETABLES

▪

REFINED FOOD

Water

Of the six components necessary for a healthy diet, water is probably the most overlooked. It contains no carbohydrates, protein or fat and therefore no calories, yet it is crucial for survival.

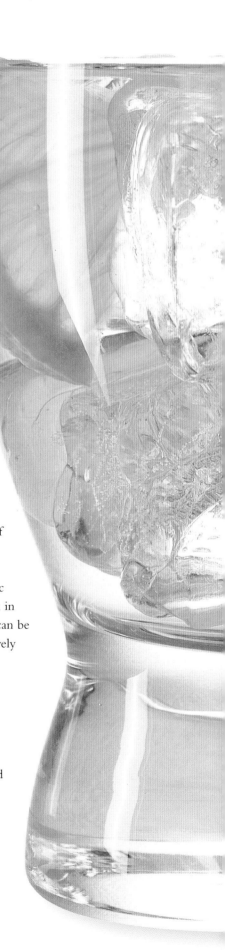

What does it do?

▪ It transports nutrients into and throughout the body, and carries waste products out again.
▪ Body temperature is stabilized by water.
▪ Water is essential for lubricating the joints, and also helps blood and other tissue fluids to flow freely.

Where is it found ?

Most of your daily intake of water is from drinks, but a significant amount is provided by food. Some foods, such as fruit and vegetables, contain a great deal of water: bananas, for example, are 75% water. In contrast, other foods, like butter, oil, biscuits and cakes, contain very little. A small amount of water is also produced by the body during the process of breaking down food for energy.

Tea, coffee and most canned fizzy drinks contain caffeine, which is a diuretic and speeds up the loss of water, increasing dehydration. Drinks that are high in sugar aren't much help either, as sugar slows down the rate at which water can be absorbed from the stomach and put to use. Even fruit juices can be deceptively high in sugar. The most efficient drink for quenching thirst is also the most straightforward: cool, preferably not iced, water.

Fluid balance

You can last without food for several weeks, but you can't survive for more than a few days without water. The amount of water you drink should balance the amount you use. An adult needs about 2.5 litres (4 pints) – around eight glasses – of water a day; in hot weather, or during exercise, you obviously need more.

Despite its importance, very few people drink enough water. By the time you feel thirsty, the dehydration process is already well under way and reaching for a drink that dehydrates makes the situation worse.

DAILY REQUIREMENT

An adult needs about 2.5 litres (4 pints) of water a day. For every 30 minutes of exercise, you should drink a glass of water.

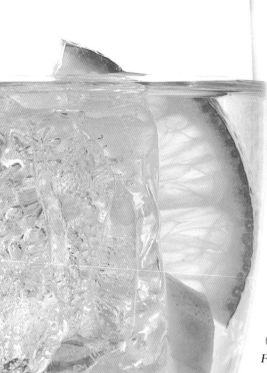

Water loss

Water is lost from the body in several ways:

As urine When protein is broken down, it leaves a waste product, called urea, that must be expelled from the body in urine. The more protein you eat, the more urea you produce. As more water is then needed to flush away the urea, if you eat large quantities of protein it can speed up dehydration.

As faeces This is made up of approximately 70% water, and accounts for a loss of about 100ml (4fl oz) of water a day. Diarrhoea or vomiting can increase the fluid loss to 5 litres (8 pints) and fluid replacement is vital.

Through the skin To maintain body temperature, you continually lose a small amount of fluid through your skin, called insensible perspiration, without ever being aware of it. You also lose over 600ml (1 pint) of water every day in sweat – exercising in hot climates can produce up to 1 litre (1.75 pints) of sweat an hour.

From the lungs When you exhale, water is lost. You only see it in very cold weather, when your breath forms a mist, but it is there whatever the temperature.

Losing water vs losing weight

Water accounts for about two-thirds of your body weight. Getting rid of this water by sweating might seem like a good way to lose weight, but losing water is not the same as losing fat: if it were, the clothes you sweat in would feel greasy, not wet.

If you stand on the scales as soon as you finish a sweaty work out, weight loss will seem to have occurred. But wait a few hours, drink a glass or two of water, and weigh yourself again: you will find that your weight is pretty much back to normal. It isn't a good idea to try to sweat yourself thin. Firstly, it won't work as any weight loss will only be temporary and, more importantly, losing even a small amount of water has serious health implications. It can affect blood pressure, temperature regulation and co-ordination and, when co-ordination is impaired, you are at risk of injury.

It is not sweat itself, but the evaporation of sweat that is the cooling mechanism of the body. In 100% humidity, the air is already saturated with as much water as it can hold, and sweat cannot evaporate. It simply rolls off the body and the cooling effect is lost.

Wearing plastic (sweat or sauna) pants affects the efficiency of sweating. By preventing the evaporation of sweat, plastic pants simply inhibit your cooling system and your body overheats. Body wraps in beauty salons work on the same principle; despite the miraculous claims for weight loss, the only thing you are losing is fluid. As soon as the body's water levels are replenished, you return to your original weight. Water loss doesn't affect body fat one little bit.

Striking a Balance

The secret of long-term weight loss does not lie in counting calories; it lies in striking a balance by making sure that the different types of food on your plate are there in the right proportions. You should get more of your calories from high-carbohydrate foods and fewer from fat.

The right balance

No diet in the world would tell you to eat as much as you like and still lose weight – if you find one that does, ignore it. There have to be a few guidelines, but these do not have to be too harsh or extreme. A diet will not work if you cannot keep it up in the long term.

A high-carbohydrate, low-fat diet provides energy and nutrients without overloading on calories but, as very few foods are 100% carbohydrates, protein or fat, you have to learn to recognize what different foods are made of, and mix and match them to create a diet that follows these guidelines:

Eat unlimited

Eat a good selection of at least five types of fruit and vegetables a day to ensure a healthy vitamin, mineral and fibre intake. Choose fresh or frozen fruit and vegetables in preference to canned, and eat them raw or lightly cooked to preserve nutrients.

Eat frequently

At least 50% of everything you eat should be

Eat sparingly

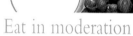
Eat in moderation

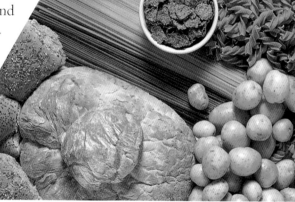
Eat frequently

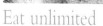
Eat unlimited

carbohydrates. If you view carbohydrates with a degree of suspicion, this might seem high. The high-protein/low-carbohydrate diet (see pages 30 – 31) of the Seventies convinced many of us that potatoes and pasta are fattening. Yet, there are plenty of examples of people who maintain lean physiques on even higher proportions of carbohydrates: in the Far East, for instance, rice traditionally provides around 80% of calories. Obesity has only recently become a problem in Japan, and it is directly related to the introduction of a Western diet that is high in protein and fat, and low in carbohydrates. Medical opinion stands firm: it is easier to store the fat you eat as body fat, than it is to store

carbohydrates as fat. To increase your carbohydrate intake, eat plenty of sugar-free breakfast cereals, bread, pasta and rice (see pages 28 – 29). Wholegrain varieties are preferable as they contain more vitamins, minerals and fibre.

Eat in moderation

Between 10 and 20% of your diet should be protein, which amounts to around two servings a day. The adult daily requirement for protein is probably lower than you think, and most of us eat more than enough protein without even trying. In developed nations, protein deficiency is virtually non-existent. Although children and pregnant women need slightly more, an adult weighing 60kg (132lb) has a daily requirement of only 45g (1½oz). In theory, 200g (7oz) of prawns would provide all the protein needed. In reality, the protein in your diet must come from a wide variety of foods to ensure a balance of essential amino acids (see pages 30 – 31). Protein is present in most foods. Meat and dairy products are high in protein but, as they can also be high in fat, choose lean meat, poultry without the skin, and low-fat cheese and milk. Dried beans, tofu and fish are also good low-fat sources of protein.

Eat sparingly

Fat should make up no more than 30% of your diet. This means foods high in fat should, for the most part, be avoided, as nearly everyone can afford to reduce the amount of fat they eat. But, however desperately you want to lose weight, do not try to cut out fat completely; it is an essential part of a balanced diet. Fat is a component of most foods, so you probably eat much more than you realize. If you are used to a high-fat diet, you may initially miss the flavour, but tastebuds can be educated; cut down gradually on the fat you eat, and you may even find you don't like it any more. Also, keep an eye on the type of fat you are eating; two-thirds of it should be unsaturated (see pages 32 – 33).

The Good Lunch Guide

Lunch is a meal we often eat on the run. Very few of us have the time to sit down for a three-course feast. This isn't necessarily a bad thing: digesting large meals often makes you feel lethargic. It makes more sense to have a lighter lunch and a reasonably sized snack (see pages 48 – 49) either side of it.

Plan ahead

If you know you are going to be away from home during the day, without access to good, healthy food, it is worth preparing your lunch in advance; fill a Thermos with soup, make a salad or sandwich, and take it with you.

Sandwiches There are so many types of bread available now, such as ciabatta, focaccia, pitta, naan, rye and soda bread, that the sandwich is no longer a boring option. Choose wholemeal bread over refined, white bread, as the fibre makes you more full. Opt for sandwiches and rolls with more bread than filling. Fillings should be low in fat, so avoid ordinary mayonnaise, butter, margarine, fatty meat or cheese. Good fillings include:
- Grilled chicken or turkey, watercress and cucumber
- Low-fat cream cheese or fromage frais with mint and sliced fresh apricots
- Low-fat hummus, grated carrot and chopped fresh coriander leaves
- Mashed banana with cottage cheese
- Low-fat mozzarella, sliced tomato and fresh basil
- Low-fat vegetable pâté.

Jacket potatoes Easy to cook, jacket potatoes provide plenty of long-term energy. They are high in fibre and contain only a trace of fat. Baked sweet potatoes are a good alternative. Fillings should be low in fat, so avoid butter and cheese, and choose from the following:
- Tuna, sweetcorn, red kidney beans, celery, spring onion and low-fat mayonnaise

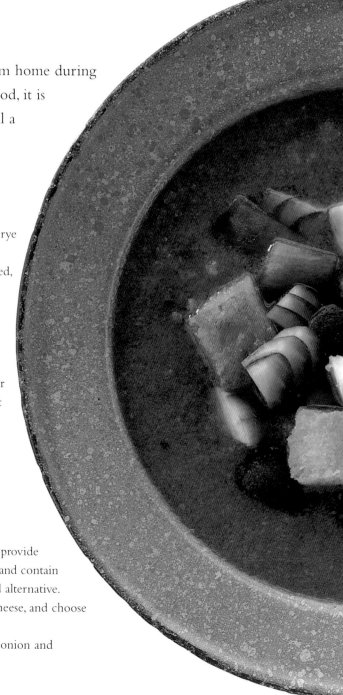

■ Baked beans spiced with Tabasco, Worcestershire sauce or chilli sauce, and chopped tomato
■ Grilled tomatoes, fresh herbs and seasoning
■ Cottage cheese with a spoonful of pesto
■ Lightly sautéed mushrooms in garlic with chopped chives and a spoonful of plain yoghurt
■ Salsa: chopped pineapple, peppers, chilli, fresh herbs and lemon juice.

Pasta

Naturally low in fat and high in carbohydrates, pasta is an excellent source of energy, but choose your sauce carefully; pasta is easily transformed into a high-fat dish by adding a cheese- or cream-based sauce. Try the following options:
■ A tomato-based sauce, with finely sliced courgettes or other raw vegetables, tossed with pasta, a small spoonful of olive oil and freshly ground black pepper
■ Pesto sauce: although it contains quite a lot of oil you need to use so little that it is not a bad choice
■ Steamed broccoli and chopped fresh chilli sautéed in a little olive oil.

Rice

Substantial and filling, rice can make a complete meal in itself when it is combined with a few other ingredients. Couscous or bulghar wheat are equally good, but brown rice has more fibre, vitamins and minerals than white rice. Try some of the following recipe ideas:
■ Add raisins and a few almonds to saffron rice
■ Stir blanched spinach leaves and diced, grilled chicken into rice that has been cooked in a stock made with garlic, cumin seeds and turmeric
■ Tuna, chopped fresh chillies and tomatoes and fresh basil stirred into cooked rice.

Soup

Serve with bread that is preferably wholemeal. Try the following combinations:
■ Cook sliced onion in a little oil, add a selection of vegetables – carrots, celery, courgettes, peppers, peas, tomatoes, potatoes – add vegetable stock, season, and cook until all the vegetables are tender. Blend to make a creamy, filling soup
■ Add canned beans – chick peas, cannellini beans, lentils – as a nutritious supplement to the above
■ Add sliced spring onions and fresh ginger to vegetable stock, pour over cooked egg noodles and sprinkle with coriander. Tofu adds a low-fat source of protein to this soup.

Salad

Although salads are a good source of vitamins and cancer-preventing nutrients, you should avoid adding fatty meat, fried croutons and avocado, which (for a fruit) is surprisingly high in fat. Similarly, salads are easily turned from a nutritious lunch into a source of fat by adding spoonfuls of dressing. The following are low-fat combinations:
■ High-carbohydrate foods like corn, kidney beans, lentils, chick peas, rice or pasta, added to chopped peppers, mushrooms, onion, celery and fresh herbs
■ Watercress or fennel mixed with sliced oranges
■ Toasted sunflower seeds or sesame seeds sprinkled over a mixed leaf salad, dressed with balsamic vinegar or lemon juice
■ Grated carrots, combined with grated fresh ginger, chives, lime juice and a few drops of sesame oil.

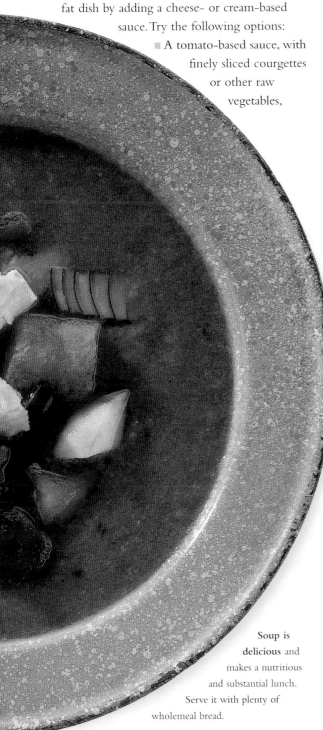

Soup is delicious and makes a nutritious and substantial lunch. Serve it with plenty of wholemeal bread.

The Good Dinner Guide

If you are cooking for yourself, it is easy to ensure that the food you eat is low in fat and high in carbohydrates. When you eat out, stick to the same criteria – avoid foods that are obviously fatty, like cream- or cheese-based sauces, or anything fried.

Meal planning

Base meals around carbohydrate foods, like pasta, rice and potatoes, rather than adopt the traditional approach, with meat as the central feature. Serve the following dishes with plenty of vegetables, grilled, steamed or roasted, or a large mixed salad:

Pasta Serve pasta with tomato or vegetable sauces, instead of high-fat meat or cream sauces. For a simple fresh tomato sauce, lightly brush halved tomatoes with a little olive oil and roast in the oven for 30 minutes. In a food processor, blend the roasted tomatoes with chopped chilli, garlic and basil leaves, and stir into cooked pasta.

Rice Brown rice is the most nutritious of all the varieties of rice and is packed wiith vitamins, minerals and fibre. You can cook brown rice in a vegetable stock with sliced dried apricots. Then fry sliced onion in a little olive oil, and add ground cumin, coriander and chilli powder. Roast cubes of pumpkin or sweet potato that have been lightly brushed with oil, and mix with the rice and spices.

Fish Fillets or steaks of fish can be given an oriental flavour: blend together fresh ginger, soy sauce, lemon juice, spring onion and five-spice powder in a food processor until they form a thick paste. Spread over the fish and grill.

Meat Choose lean cuts of meat and trim off any obvious fat before cooking. Use a cooking method that allows the fat to drain away – grilling or roasting, rather than frying. Dab meat with kitchen towels to soak up any excess fat after cooking. Marinades add flavour to meat without adding a lot of extra fat. For a Moroccan-inspired marinade, combine lemon juice with chilli powder, cumin, paprika and a splash of olive oil. Marinate cubed lean lamb, chicken, or fish for at least one hour before grilling.

Poultry Choose grilled chicken or turkey. Much of the fat in poultry lies under and in the skin, so remove it before cooking to prevent the fat seeping into the flesh as it cooks. The marinades for meat or fish are equally good with poultry.

Pizza This can make a well-balanced meal, especially when the crust is thick or deep-pan; it is the pizza topping that can be a problem. Avoid meat, keep high-fat cheese to a minimum, and choose vegetable-based toppings instead. Top a pizza base with a fresh tomato sauce or a thin layer of pesto sauce or olive paste, and add thinly sliced mushrooms, peppers, tomatoes and garlic. Sprinkle with fresh or dried oregano or fresh basil. Drizzle with olive oil, if desired, and bake in the oven until crisp and golden.

Vegetables Most of us do not eat enough vegetables, yet they contain vital vitamins and minerals, and they are very low in fat. Allow vegetables to form the central part of a meal: stuff peppers or aubergines with a mix of onions, peppers, courgettes, herbs and tomatoes cooked in a little olive oil. Bake in the oven for one hour and serve with rice. For variety, add tuna, sweetcorn, chick peas or black-eye beans. Puréed vegetables also make simple and nutritious sauces and soups.

Potatoes To replace chips, cut potatoes into wedge shapes, lay on a baking tray, season, and drizzle with a little olive oil. Bake in the oven for one hour, until golden. Alternatively, thinly slice potatoes and combine with sliced onion, tomato, fresh rosemary and garlic in a baking dish. Pour over some vegetable stock, cover with foil, and bake in the oven for one hour.

Room for dessert

If you eat a main course that is high in carbohydrates, you will probably find that you do not have room for dessert. However, if you are still hungry, here are some healthy options:

▪ Fresh fruit – melon, kiwi fruit, grapes
▪ Low-fat yoghurt mixed with fruit and sunflower seeds, or sweetened with a little honey
▪ Baked apple stuffed with raisins, dates or dried apricots and a little honey
▪ Low-fat rice pudding, sprinkled with grated nutmeg
▪ Puréed mango or pineapple mixed into plain yoghurt or low-fat fromage frais
▪ Fruit purée – for a simple fruit sauce, blend frozen raspberries and strawberries in a liquidizer (add a little caster sugar if the fruit is very tart). Pass the purée through a sieve to remove the seeds, and serve warm or cold with low-fat yoghurt or fruit sorbet
▪ Stewed dried fruit – figs, dates, apricots, apples, sultanas, peaches and pears
▪ Meringues with fruit and low-fat fromage frais.

Be imaginative in your use of vegetables – they can form the central part of a meal.

47

The Good Snack Guide

The point of "snacking" is to bridge the gap between main meals and keep blood sugar levels constant. When your blood sugar fluctuates, so does your energy. To avoid this, you should snack on foods where the calories come from complex carbohydrates, not from fat.

Healthy snacks

Many snack foods are very high in fat. We all underestimate how much we eat, and it is easy to overlook the odd handful of peanuts now and then, but that odd handful can add considerably to the total amount of fat you eat. To avoid temptation, create a "safe" environment in your home or work-place by surrounding yourself with plenty of low-fat foods to snack on. If you feel an irresistible craving for something indulgent, it's probably better to go for a sweet treat rather than a fatty one.

Fruit The perfect snack food, fruit even comes ready-wrapped. Where fruit is concerned, there are no restrictions; no fruit (except avocado) is more fattening than any other. Fruit contains practically no fat at all. It is mainly carbohydrates, at least 50% water, and is also high in vitamins.

Dried fruit A compact source of sweetness as well as vitamins and minerals, dried fruit also provides valuable fibre. Dried apricots, raisins, prunes and sultanas are high in iron and potassium.

Raw vegetables Often overlooked as a snack food, this is probably because most vegetables need some preparation before they are eaten. In fact, once they are washed, many vegetables can be eaten raw. They are a good source of carbohydrates, and contain plenty of vitamins, minerals and fibre.

Pitta bread Low-fat hummus, salad, or grilled vegetables mixed with a little pesto sauce or olive tapenade, make delicious fillings for pitta bread.

Rice cakes Nibble them plain, or top with absolutely anything – vegetables, fresh fruit, jam or cottage cheese.

English muffins and scones These are a healthy source of carbohydrates, but are often turned into a high-fat snack by adding butter and cream. Muffins and scones have a natural sweetness, so try them on their own, or top them with soft fruit, such as strawberries, raspberries or blueberries, and a spoonful of low-fat Greek yoghurt.

Sandwiches and rolls make an excellent high-carbohydrate snack.

If you really crave butter, try to switch to a low-fat spread. These contain about half the fat of butter, but choose one that is unhydrogenated (see page 33), as it is much better for your health.

Bagels Versatile and convenient, bagels can be bought in either sweet or savoury varieties. Onion or pumpernickel bagels can be eaten with a thin layer of low-fat cream cheese, cottage cheese with chives or spring onion, or low-fat vegetable pâté. Sweet bagels, like cinnamon and raisin, do not need much in the way of topping and are perfect toasted with sliced banana or low-sugar, high-fruit jam.

Pretzels An excellent source of carbohydrates, but avoid those that are heavily coated in salt.

Popcorn A healthy snack, as long as the popcorn is not coated with oil, butter or salt. Try making popcorn yourself and flavouring it with paprika, soy sauce, Tabasco or, for a sweet alternative, cinnamon or nutmeg. Avoid the ready-made, caramel-coated variety: the coating is pure refined sugar.

Low-fat biscuits Usually lower in fat than normal biscuits, but check the label as many low-fat biscuits are loaded with refined sugar to compensate for the lack of taste. The calories are often just as high – they just come from a different source. Choose biscuits that are as close to crackers as possible.

Sandwiches An excellent high-carbohydrate snack, as long as the filling is low in fat. For filling ideas, see pages 44 – 45.

Breadsticks These can be eaten on their own, or dipped into low-fat hummus or tzatziki.

Yoghurt All yoghurt is made with milk, but this is often where the similarity ends. It can be made with whole or skimmed milk and sometimes has added sugar, cream or other flavourings. Look at the label, as the fat content of yoghurt can vary from 0.2g (0.01oz) per 100g (3.6oz) in low-fat yoghurt to 9g (0.3oz) per 100g (3.6oz) in full-fat Greek yoghurt. Plain yoghurt can be flavoured with fresh or dried fruit, fruit purée, nutmeg, cinnamon, or used as a low-fat salad dressing. Low-fat fromage frais and crème fraîche are now also widely available.

49

Total Fitness Plan

I am no stranger to exercise – I have been

dancing for most of my life – but the first time

I decided to exercise for *fitness*, I felt as if I was

gatecrashing a private party.

Fitness has become a bit exclusive: you probably think you

have to buy the right gear, join a gym, or hire a personal

trainer if you're serious about getting fit.

In fact you don't need to do any of these things. All you

need to get fit is a good pair of trainers, the right advice,

and a healthy dose of determination. It will all feel a little

strange at first, but bear in mind an old Norwegian

saying: "The mile across the doorstep is the longest".

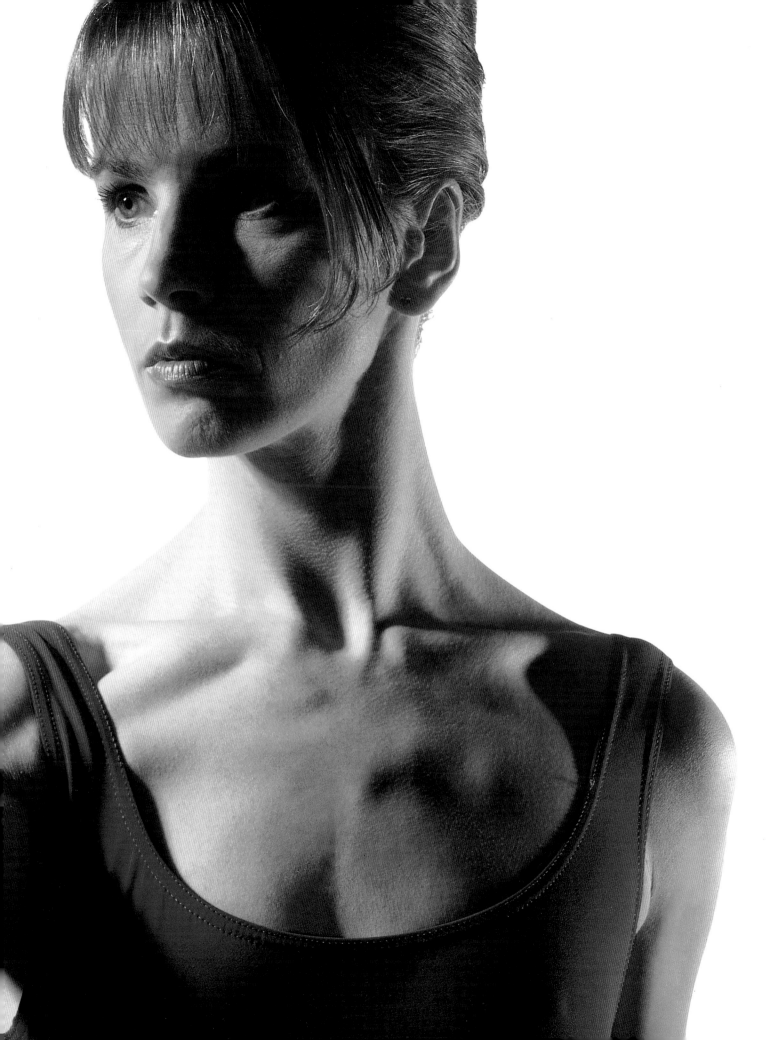

Getting the Right Gear

There are no hard and fast rules about what to wear when you exercise, unless you intend to take up competitive athletics. In some ways, the most important thing is to feel comfortable. However, as all physical exercise involves sweating – you're going to get wet – some clothes are more suitable than others.

Keeping warm, staying cool

The evaporation of sweat is the body's cooling mechanism. In windy weather, when evaporation is rapid, you risk cooling down too much. The trick is to wear "breathable" clothing that allows sweat to evaporate yet keeps you warm throughout your work out (see side bar). Always wear socks: the Achilles' tendon is never very warm, and a cold tendon is at risk of injury. There is also a practical concern – without socks, sweat quickly rots shoes.

WARM WEATHER

Shorts or track pants and a loose T-shirt.

This is the only weather when shorts are suitable: sweating limbs are best covered up. In intense sunshine, use a sweat-resistant sunscreen to avoid getting burnt.

COOL WEATHER

Track-pants and a top of moisture-transporting fabric, such as polypropylene.

You can add a sweatshirt, and (if it's windy) a breathable windbreaker.

COLD WEATHER

Moisture-transporting fabric on the legs and upper body.

You can cover this with track-pants and a thin wool layer, like an old sweater. You may need a breathable windbreaker, gloves, and even a woollen hat.

Trainers

To avoid the risk of injury, you should always wear good shoes: this may be the one expense necessary before you can begin. Appropriate shoes are especially important if you plan on jogging.

Bike

For general training, choose a "hybrid" bike. Mountain bikes are really for serious off-road cycling, although "slick" tyres will make them smoother for road use.

Helmet

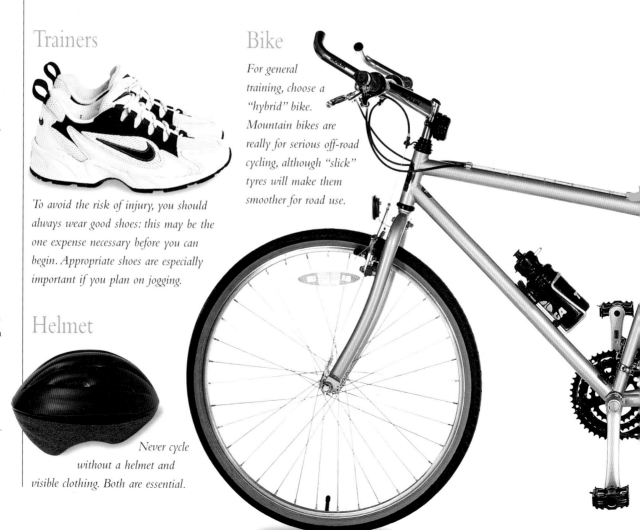

Never cycle without a helmet and visible clothing. Both are essential.

A firm footing

If you're not used to physical activity, exercise will put an unfamiliar strain on your joints, muscles and tendons. It is vital that you give them as much support as possible by wearing the best trainers that you can afford; don't be tempted to go out in your old school plimsolls (hang on to them though, they provide some valuable information).

Go to a specialist shop and ask for a shoe designed to support your particular type of feet. Take your old shoes with you – they will provide clues as to the sort of trainers you should buy as a replacement.

There are basically three types of feet (see right): flat, "pronating" feet that roll inward, high-arched "supinating" feet that roll outward, and "neutral" feet that are more or less straight. When the feet roll either way, the shoes have to compensate. Pronating feet need "straight-lasted" trainers with good arch- and medial support. Supinating feet need trainers with good arch- and lateral support, and with especially

good shock absorbency, as these feet can be rather rigid. All trainers should be snug, but not tight, and should have good shock absorbency. Unless you intend to run only on dry pavements, avoid smooth-soled shoes, which will be slippery in wet or muddy conditions. Try several pairs before you decide – don't just go for the ones with the best colour scheme. Trainers should be chosen with the feet, not the eyes.

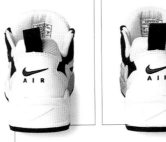

Pronating feet will wear trainers out along here

Supinating feet will wear trainers out along here

WIND CHILL

However warm the temperature, wind speed can have a dramatic effect on how warm you feel. This is known as the "wind-chill" factor. Cyclists should pay particular attention to wind chill, as cycling into the wind increases its cooling effect.

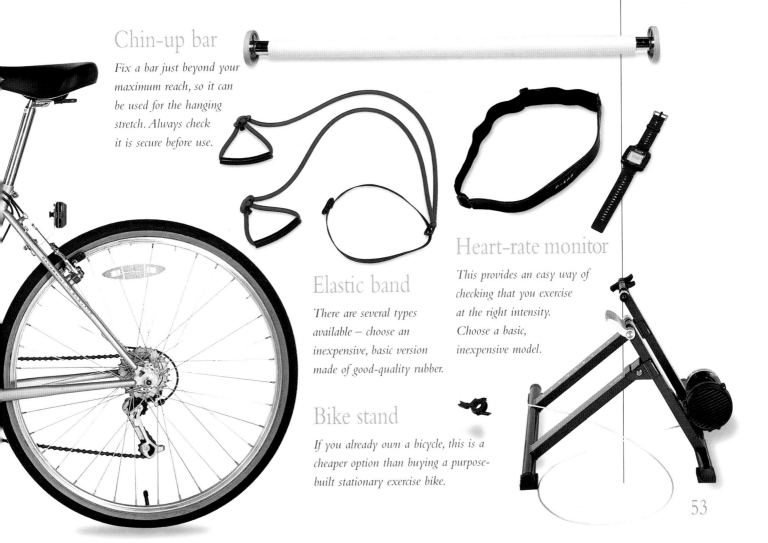

Chin-up bar

Fix a bar just beyond your maximum reach, so it can be used for the hanging stretch. Always check it is secure before use.

Elastic band

There are several types available – choose an inexpensive, basic version made of good-quality rubber.

Bike stand

If you already own a bicycle, this is a cheaper option than buying a purpose-built stationary exercise bike.

Heart-rate monitor

This provides an easy way of checking that you exercise at the right intensity. Choose a basic, inexpensive model.

When To Exercise

It doesn't matter what time of the day you exercise. Although some experts claim that a morning work out raises the metabolic rate and keeps it elevated for the rest of the day, others have found no evidence of any "after burning" effect. Ultimately, it comes down to practicalities. You have to find a space in the day that suits you.

Eating and exercise

Fitting exercise around meal times requires a little planning. You obviously don't want to work out feeling hungry, nor do you want to feel bloated. When you eat is almost as important as what you eat. If you are exercising primarily to burn fat, it is especially important that you do not eat just beforehand. In response to food, the pancreas releases the hormone insulin, which temporarily prevents fat being used as a source of energy.

A question of timing

Digesting a large meal takes several hours, and during this time you won't feel very energetic. There are two reasons for this: firstly, blood is diverted to the stomach to digest the food, so there is less blood available to carry oxygen to the muscles. Secondly, the pancreas releases insulin, and this may make you feel lethargic. The brain requires a constant level of sugar in the blood, and insulin helps to regulate this. When food is digested, the sugar it contains is absorbed into the bloodstream, and the blood-sugar level increases. To counter this, insulin is released to "push" this sugar into the muscles and liver. The consequent drop in blood sugar may bring about a temporary feeling of tiredness. Refined sugar, which releases its energy in one great surge, causes the insulin to overcompensate, which can lead to bouts of dizziness.

You should allow at least two hours between eating and exercise so that you aren't affected by any dips in energy levels. If you've eaten sufficient carbohydrates, you'll have plenty of stored energy available. Work outs lasting less than 90 minutes rely entirely on stored fuel; it's only when you exercise for longer than this that food eaten immediately before or during exercise starts to provide energy.

If you choose to work out first thing in the morning, it can be difficult to fit in breakfast beforehand. Have some fruit or a glass of fruit juice 30 minutes before you start; this will be enough to get you going. Be sure to eat breakfast afterwards.

Energy drinks

Marketing men are a little unscrupulous when they use the word "energy", failing to mention that "low calorie" means low energy, or that "energy" drinks provide energy because they are high in calories.

If you are ill, energy drinks can be very useful, and if you're running a marathon, they can be a lifeline. But if your main objective is to burn fat, energy drinks may not be a good idea, as the sugar content causes the pancreas to produce insulin. While the insulin level in the blood is high, fat cannot be used for energy. If you feel listless or lethargic, take a look at your diet and your lifestyle. Don't imagine you can open a bottle and instantly solve the problem.

The Pre-exercise Plan

Unless you're very fit, it's not a good idea to launch into exercise without a little preparation. Most importantly, leaping directly from the sofa to a 30-minute work out puts you at risk of injury. Even if you escape this, you will ache so much from the unfamiliar activity that you would probably give up on day two.

The three starting levels

Depending on your general fitness, your body takes at least two weeks to adjust to any increase in activity. During this time, the overriding concern is injury prevention. Don't worry that you're not burning fat: it is more important to strengthen your muscles, tendons and ligaments so that you can eventually follow the Total Fitness Plan without interruption from injury. Be sure to complete Level 3 before you move on to the fitness plan.

Where to begin

Every novice exerciser starts from a different level – be honest with yourself, and choose the one that best describes your general fitness. Finish each fitness session with a light stretch (see pages 58 – 59). When you have completed one level, move on to the next. Once you have completed all three, you are ready to start the Total Fitness Plan.

It's also a good idea to start increasing your general level of activity during the day. This will give a much needed boost to your metabolism. Any of the following can be easily incorporated into your daily routine:

- Cycle or walk to work.
- If it is not possible to walk all the way, park further from the office, and walk the last couple of miles.
- Get off the bus or tube a few stops early. You might also save money!
- Walk up stairs instead of taking the lift or the escalator.
- Don't use the car for short trips – walk them instead.

LEVEL 1
YEARS OF NEGLECT

Unable to walk up a flight of stairs without stopping.
Two weeks of the following:

- *45 seconds of slow walking*
- *15 seconds of fast walking*

Alternate between these for 5 minutes daily. Add 1 minute every second day. Finish each session with the light stretch.

LEVEL 2
UNFIT

Out of breath after climbing a flight of stairs.
Two weeks of the following:

- *1 minute of slow walking*
- *1 minute of fast walking*

Alternate between these for 10 minutes daily. Add 1 minute every second day. Finish each session with the light stretch.

LEVEL 3
FAIRLY FIT

No restrictions in day-to-day activity.
Two weeks of the following:

- *1 minute of slow walking*
- *30 seconds of easy jogging*

Alternate between these for 10 minutes daily. Add 1 minute every second day. Finish each session with the light stretch.

Aerobic Exercise

The aerobic element is the part of your work out designed to burn fat. To achieve this effectively, you have to keep it up for at least 20 minutes, at 60 – 70% of your heart's maximum capacity. Only then, when exercise is of the right intensity and duration, will the energy you use come from body fat.

Starting out

When you begin, you may find that brisk walking is enough to raise the heart rate to 60 – 70% of its capacity, especially if you are not used to exercise. As you get fitter, your heart, like the rest of your muscles, will become stronger, and you will need to increase the pace to push your heart rate to the right level.

Staying in the target zone

As exercise has to be of the right intensity to burn fat, it is important to work out your personal target zone before you start (see pages 22 – 23), and to keep within it. At first, you need to take your pulse at regular intervals to check that your heart is working at the right level. After a while, you will begin to recognize this level, using pace and breathing as indicators, and you won't need to test it quite so often. If you want to be really sure that you are within your target zone, you can buy a heart rate monitor (see page 53).

A defining characteristic of aerobic exercise is that it can be sustained for long periods of time. If you can't keep going, it's probably because you've pushed your heart rate too high. Slow down to a walking pace, and gradually speed up again when it has returned to the target level. Whatever you do, to burn a signficant amount of fat, you must keep going for at least 20 minutes.

If at first you find it difficult to train at a consistent pace for 20 – 30 minutes, try interval training (see tint box, below). Alternating between walking and jogging is the easiest form of interval training and you can use the same formula for any type of activity. This type of training is often more enjoyable, and can also be gentler on the joints than keeping a steady pace.

INTERVAL TRAINING

- *Once you have warmed up, jog until your heart rate reaches 70% of your maximum capacity (see pages 22 – 23).*
- *Slow down the pace to a walk until the heart rate drops to 60% of its maximum.*
- *Step up the pace until the heart rate reaches 70% again.*
- *Continue to alternate between the two for the duration of your work out.*

Choosing your exercise

There are several types of aerobic exercise, and you can choose whichever you like. Your heart doesn't know what type of exercise you are doing; it will only register the fact that your muscles require more oxygen. The "ideal" exercise for burning fat is the one that suits you best, although varying the activity from time to time will reduce the risk of over-using specific joints.

Brisk walking Probably the perfect exercise when you first start out, especially if you're very overweight. It's safe, familiar, low in impact and easy to keep up.

Cross-country skiing If you have access to snow, this is an excellent form of exercise. Cross-country skiers are regularly shown to have the highest fitness levels of all athletes, and relatively low levels of body fat. Cross-country skiing uses all the major muscle groups in the arms and legs, and is very low in impact. Many gyms have exercise machines that simulate cross-country skiing.

Cycling A good alternative to jogging. When cycling, the body weight is supported, so it's gentler on the joints. It does require some equipment – a helmet and visible clothing – but lots of people already own a bike. You do need to be mindful of the wind-chill factor. In bad weather, you can cycle indoors with the aid of a bike stand, which converts your bicycle into a stationary exercise bike (see page 53). These are quite inexpensive and can be bought at a good cycling shop.

Back Extensions

This exercise targets most of the muscles in the back, especially the erector spinae muscles which run prominently down both sides of the spine. Back extensions are important because they balance the strength of the abdominals and improve posture. If either the back or abdominal muscle groups are weak, there is a risk of lower back pain and injury.

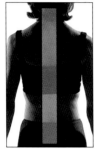

THE ERECTOR SPINAE MUSCLES are attached to each vertebra down the spine, from the base of the skull to the pelvis.

1 ***Lie face down***, *flat on the floor, with your arms stretched straight out above your head.*

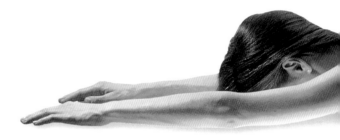

2 ***First tighten your buttock muscles,*** *then lift your arms and legs steadily, so that your nose and knees are just off the ground. Hold this position for a count of 3, then gently lower your body. Relax for a count of 3, then repeat. Start with 2 sets of 3 lifts, building up to 3 sets of 10 lifts.*

Lift both arms and legs at a steady rate

Do not raise the head above the arms

CAUTION

Always tighten the buttocks before commencing Step 2, to protect the lower back.

Do not lift the back or the legs too high off the ground.

The upper body lifts until the nose is just off the ground

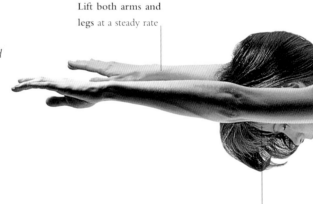

"*Back extensions*

will help to give you a dancer's

strength in your back."

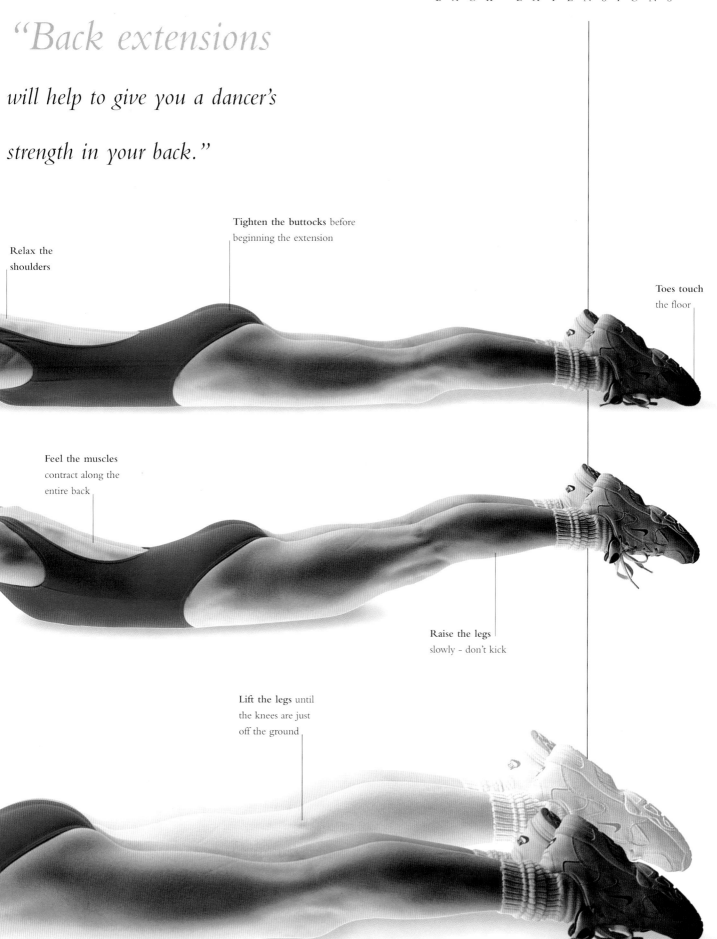

Relax the
shoulders

Tighten the buttocks before
beginning the extension

Toes touch
the floor

Feel the muscles
contract along the
entire back

Raise the legs
slowly - don't kick

Lift the legs until
the knees are just
off the ground

67

Chair Dips

Chair dips offer an excellent alternative to the more usual push-ups as they work a wider combination of muscles. This is a very safe way of exercising the latissimus dorsi in the back, as well as the triceps and pectorals, because it provides some traction for the spine. Chair dips will improve muscle tone in the torso, and help firm the back of the upper arms.

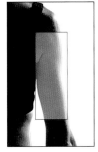

THE TRICEPS MUSCLE is situated along the back of the upper arm, and crosses both the shoulder-joint and the elbow.

1 *Support yourself* with both hands on the seat of a chair, so that your arms are slightly behind you. Suspend your weight on both arms and stretch your legs out in front of you.

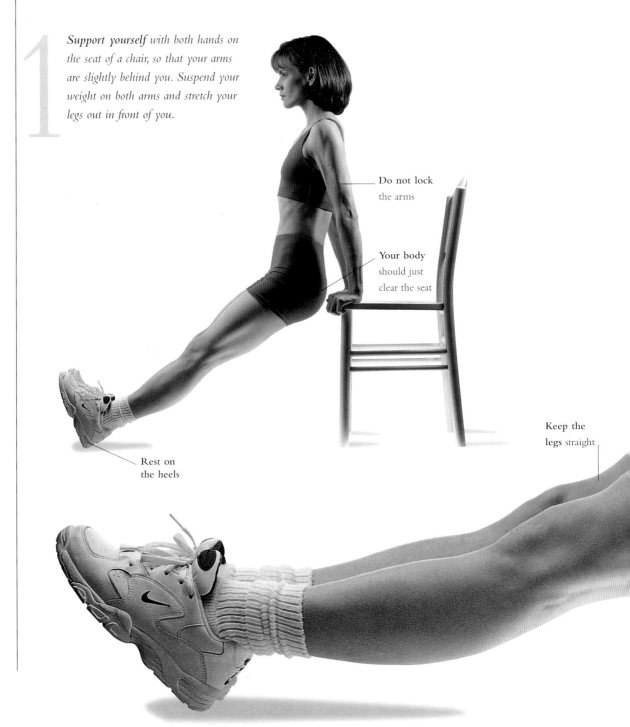

Do not lock the arms

Your body should just clear the seat

Keep the legs straight

Rest on the heels

CAUTION

Do not lower yourself too far at first, or you might strain the shoulder joint.

68

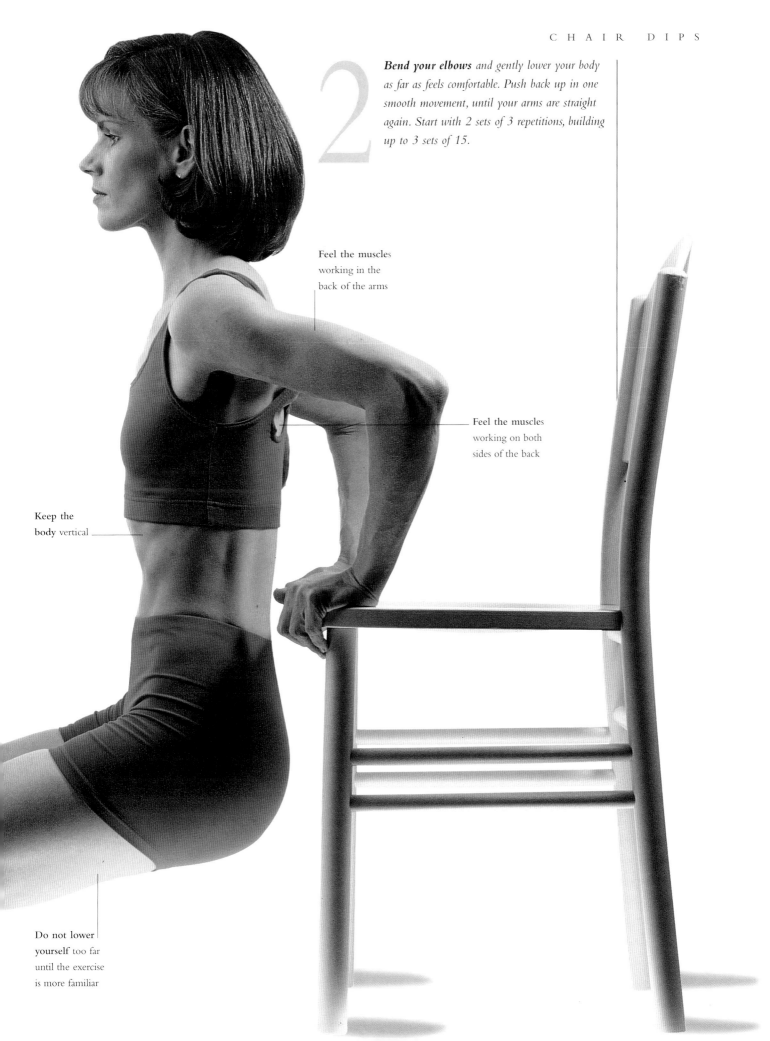

2

Bend your elbows and gently lower your body as far as feels comfortable. Push back up in one smooth movement, until your arms are straight again. Start with 2 sets of 3 repetitions, building up to 3 sets of 15.

Feel the muscles working in the back of the arms

Feel the muscles working on both sides of the back

Keep the **body** vertical

Do not lower yourself too far until the exercise is more familiar

Hamstrings

Strong and flexible hamstrings contribute to good posture, and work together with the abdominals to protect the lower back. Since most aerobic exercise, such as running and cycling, strengthens the quadriceps at the front of the thigh, it is important to balance this with selective training of the hamstrings.

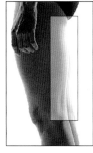

THE HAMSTRINGS is the collective name for the group of muscles in the back of the thigh. They originate at the back of the pelvis and attach below the knee.

Double hamstring

1 *Lie flat on the floor with your arms at your sides for support. Place both heels of your feet on the seat of a chair, with your knees bent at right-angles.*

Spread the arms slightly for stability

Knees and hips are bent at a 90° angle

2 *Lift your pelvis high off the floor by pushing your weight down onto your heels. Hold the position briefly.*

Feet rest on the heels

3 *Move your pelvis up and down, without letting your bottom touch the ground. Rest and repeat. Start with 2 sets of 3 repetitions, building up to 3 sets of 7.*

Keep the arms flat on the ground

Do not let the bottom touch the floor

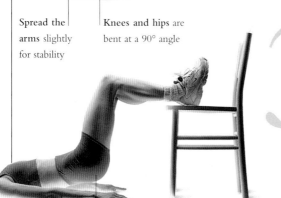

CAUTION

This is quite a tough exercise. Do not attempt too many repetitions until accustomed to it.

One-legged hamstring

You can progress to this exercise once you are able to complete the double hamstring with ease. Lie as before, but with your right heel on the seat of the chair and your left leg pointing upward. Lift your pelvis high off the floor by pushing down through your right heel, and move up and down as before, without letting your body touch the ground. Lower yourself down and repeat with your other leg. Start with 2 sets of 6 repetitions, building up to 3 sets of 14.

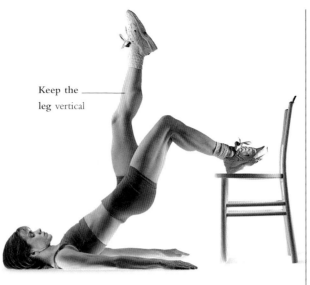

Keep the leg vertical

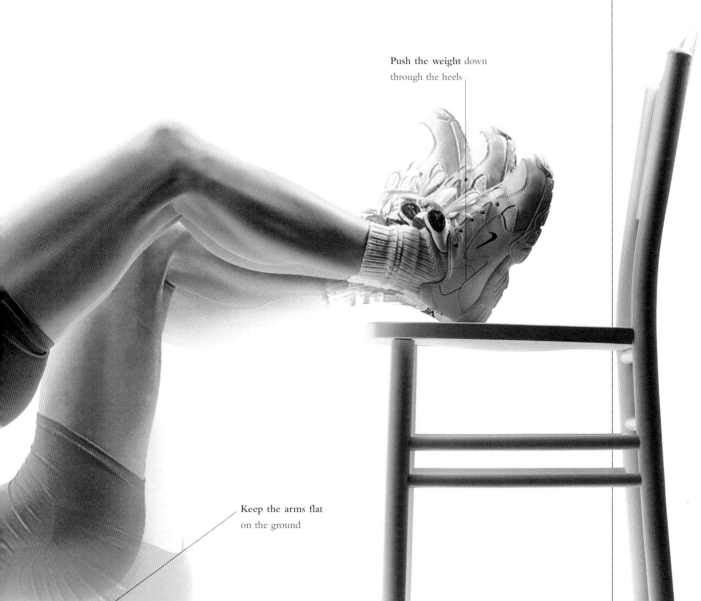

Push the weight down through the heels

Keep the arms flat on the ground

Biceps

This exercise can be performed in any one of three ways. The chin-up works the biceps and the brachialis muscles, while the inclined chin-up and the arm-curl, with its elastic resistance, offer an easier alternative which women may find easier to execute. For the chin-up, you will need a bar or a tree branch, and for the arm-curl you will need an elastic exercise band (see page 52).

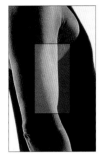

THE BICEPS and THE BRACHIALIS MUSCLES oppose the TRICEPS. Together, they provide bulk and strength in the upper arm.

Chin-up

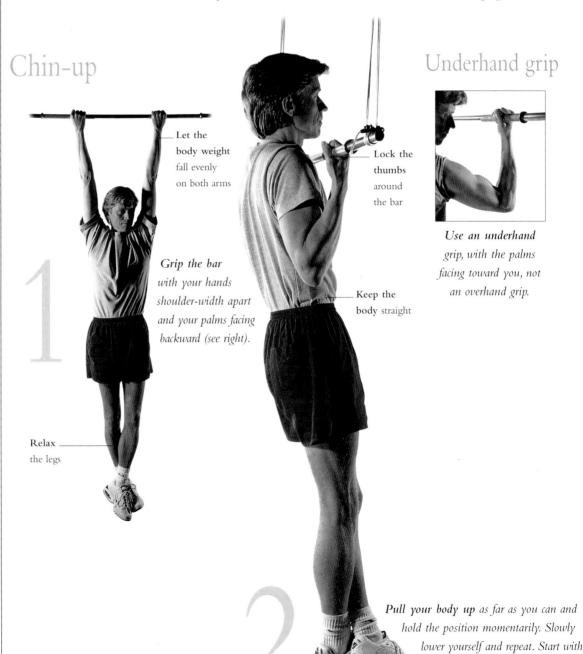

1

Let the **body weight** fall evenly on both arms

Grip the bar with your hands shoulder-width apart and your palms facing backward (see right).

Relax the legs

Lock the thumbs around the bar

Keep the **body** straight

Underhand grip

Use an underhand grip, with the palms facing toward you, not an overhand grip.

2

Pull your body up as far as you can and hold the position momentarily. Slowly lower yourself and repeat. Start with 2 sets of 2 repetitions, building up to 3 sets of 7 repetitions.

CAUTION

If the chin-up feels too hard, do arm-curls until you have increased your strength.

Inclined chin-up

1 *Fix the bar* at waist height. Grasp it with an underhand grip (see left), hands shoulder-width apart, keeping your body straight and your heels on the ground.

Keep the body straight

Heels are hip-width apart

Check that the body is in line

2 *Pull yourself up* as high as possible and hold momentarily before slowly lowering yourself. Start with 2 sets of 2 repetitions, building up to 3 sets of 7 repetitions.

Arm-curl

1 *Place your right foot* slightly in front of your left and fix the elastic beneath it. Hold the elastic in your right hand, with your elbow bent and the elastic tight enough to give slight resistance.

Keep the legs apart for stability

Elastic exercise band

Adjust elastic tension so that the repetitions are just possible

Hold the back straight

Ensure that the elbow remains close to the body

2 *Bend your elbow* and pull the elastic up to your shoulder. Hold the position briefly, before slowly lowering your arm. Start with 2 sets of 6 repetitions on each arm, building up to 3 sets of 10 repetitions.

CAUTION

Do not let the elastic slip from beneath the foot.

73

Arabesque

This is one of the most common positions in ballet. Here, it is borrowed from the dance class and adapted for use in strength training. Ballet technique is not always appropriate for non-dancers, but the combination of turn-out and lift in the arabesque is particularly effective in working the gluteal muscles and firming the buttocks.

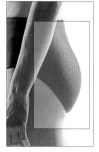

THE GLUTEAL MUSCLES make up the bulk of the buttocks. They connect the pelvis and the femur bone in the thigh.

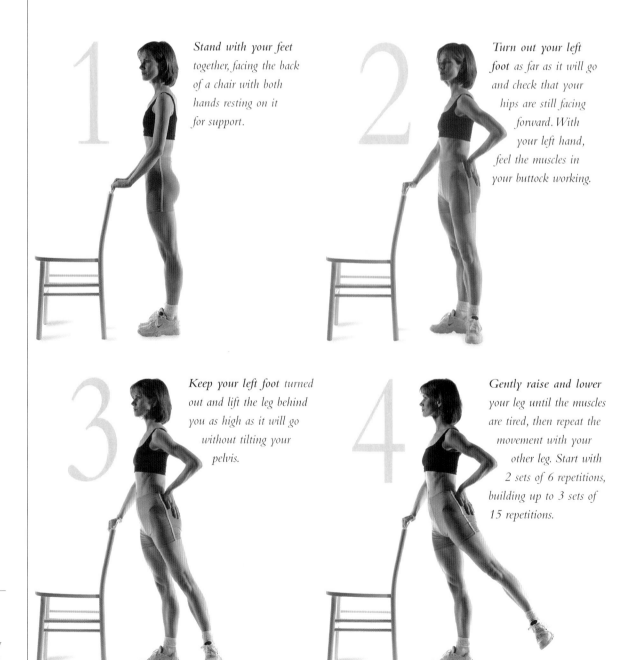

1 *Stand with your feet together, facing the back of a chair with both hands resting on it for support.*

2 *Turn out your left foot as far as it will go and check that your hips are still facing forward. With your left hand, feel the muscles in your buttock working.*

3 *Keep your left foot turned out and lift the leg behind you as high as it will go without tilting your pelvis.*

4 *Gently raise and lower your leg until the muscles are tired, then repeat the movement with your other leg. Start with 2 sets of 6 repetitions, building up to 3 sets of 15 repetitions.*

CAUTION

Do not lift the foot too high, or you may strain the lower back.

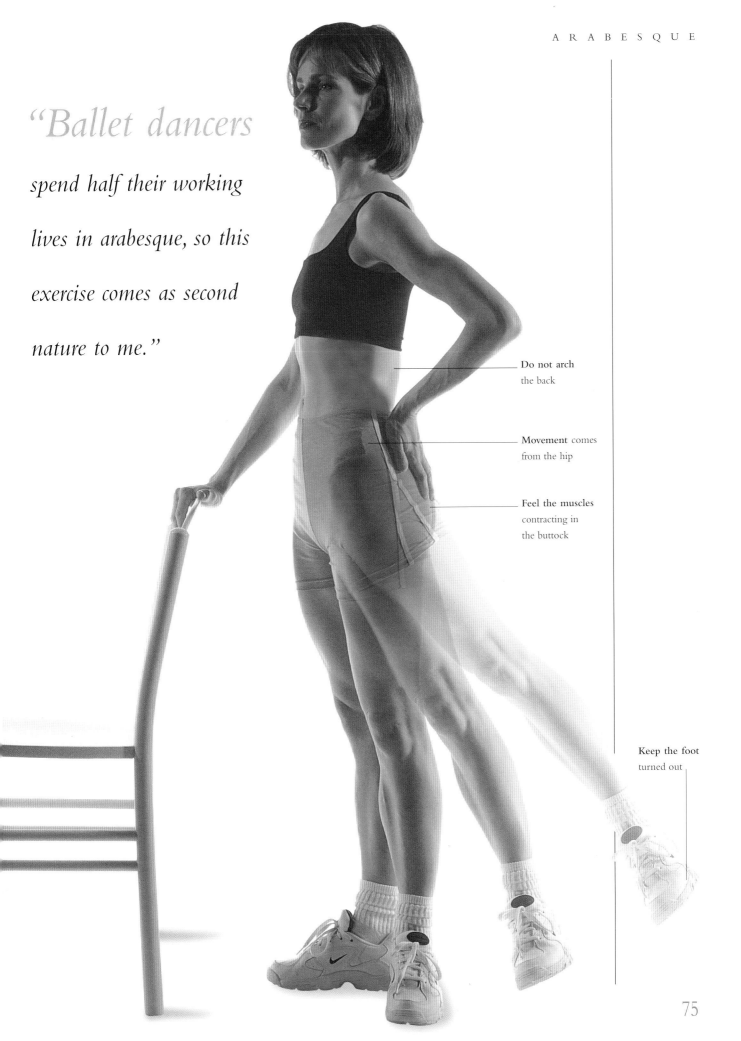

"Ballet dancers spend half their working lives in arabesque, so this exercise comes as second nature to me."

Do not arch
the back

Movement comes
from the hip

Feel the muscles
contracting in
the buttock

Keep the foot
turned out

Inner Thigh

The adductors are the muscles on the inside of the thighs that bring the legs together – you feel them work when you cross one leg over the other. This exercise has a strong aesthetic factor, as it helps to firm the inner thighs. It also develops the specific strength needed in sports such as football, skiing and rollerblading.

THE ADDUCTOR MUSCLES stretch between the knee and the pelvis, on the inside of the thigh.

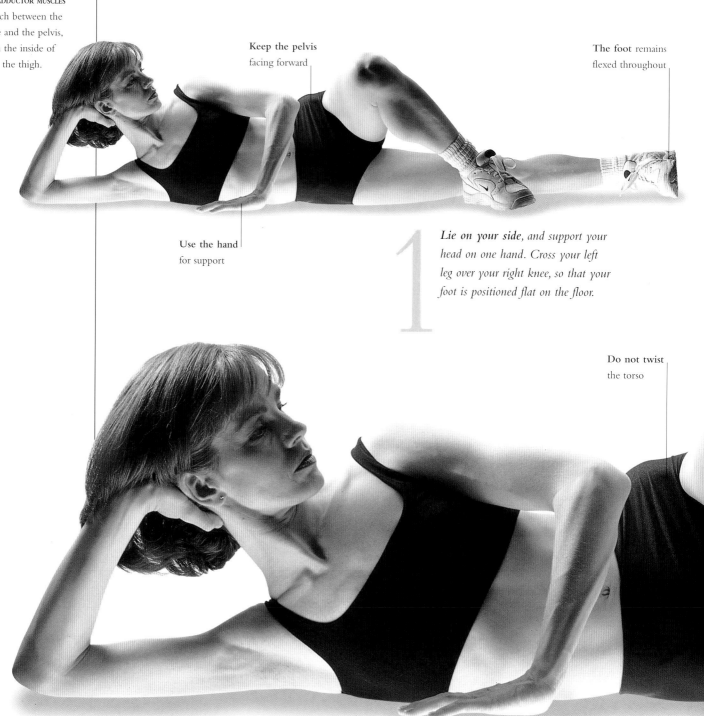

Keep the pelvis facing forward

The foot remains flexed throughout

Use the hand for support

1 *Lie on your side, and support your head on one hand. Cross your left leg over your right knee, so that your foot is positioned flat on the floor.*

Do not twist the torso

"*Feel the muscles*

working by resting your hand on

your leg from time to time."

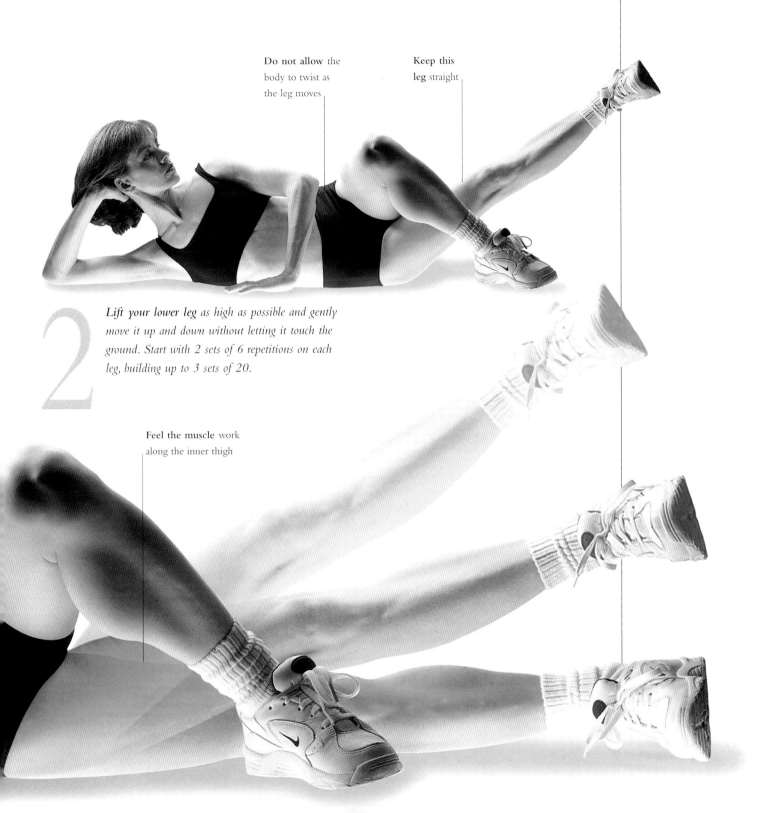

Do not allow the body to twist as the leg moves

Keep this leg straight

2

Lift your lower leg as high as possible and gently move it up and down without letting it touch the ground. Start with 2 sets of 6 repetitions on each leg, building up to 3 sets of 20.

Feel the muscle work along the inner thigh

Deltoid

A large, triangular muscle, the deltoid covers the shoulder and is used to lift the arm. By lifting the arm sideways, against elastic resistance, you work as much of the muscle as possible in one movement. This exercise tones the shoulders, strengthens the arms, and improves the look of the upper body. You will need an elastic exercise band (see pages 52 – 53).

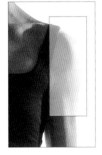

THE DELTOID MUSCLE originates from the collar bone and shoulder blade and attaches to the humerus, the bone of the upper arm.

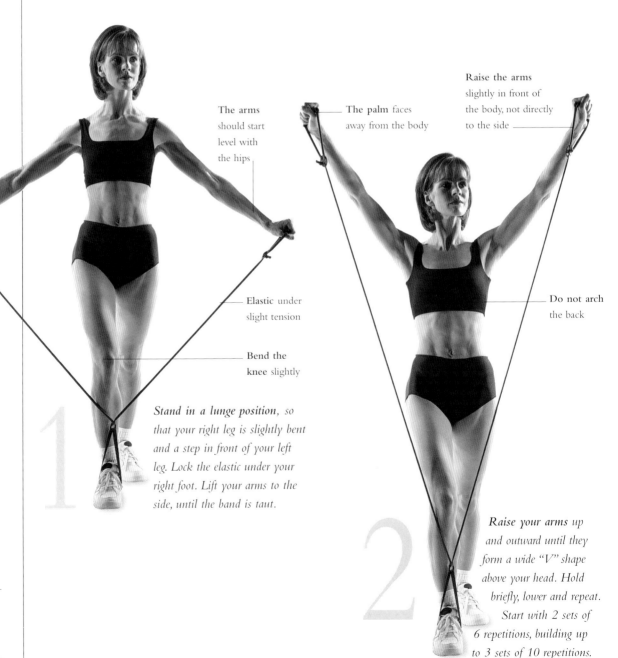

The arms should start level with the hips

The palm faces away from the body

Raise the arms slightly in front of the body, not directly to the side

Elastic under slight tension

Bend the knee slightly

Do not arch the back

Stand in a lunge position, so that your right leg is slightly bent and a step in front of your left leg. Lock the elastic under your right foot. Lift your arms to the side, until the band is taut.

Raise your arms up and outward until they form a wide "V" shape above your head. Hold briefly, lower and repeat. Start with 2 sets of 6 repetitions, building up to 3 sets of 10 repetitions.

CAUTION

Check that the elastic does not slip.

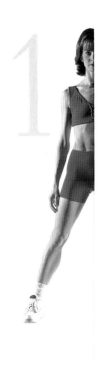

Inne

of muscles o

A healthy bac

and if the addu

they can limit m

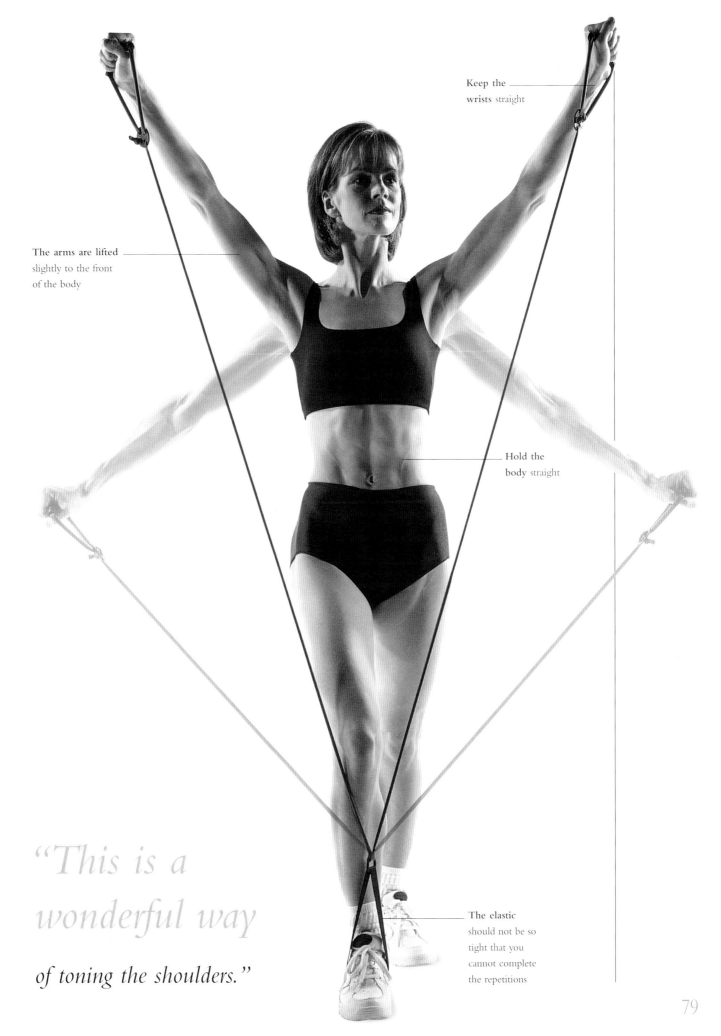

The arms are lifted
slightly to the front
of the body

Keep the
wrists straight

Hold the
body straight

The elastic
should not be so
tight that you
cannot complete
the repetitions

"This is a
wonderful way

of toning the shoulders."

St Hip Flexor

The psoas muscle, commonly called the hip flexor, lifts the leg in front of the body – an action used, for instance, in running and walking. Due to its complex relationship with the hip and spine, it rarely gets to stretch out fully. A tight psoas pulls on the lower spine, contributing to back pain. Combining a flexible psoas with strong abdominal muscles protects the lower back.

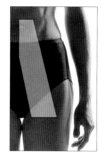

THE PSOAS MUSCLE
(the "p" is silent)
runs between the
femur, or thigh bone,
and the lower spine.

THE STRETCHES

Do each stretch on
both sides of the body,
then repeat.

■

INNER THIGH

■

HIP FLEXOR

■

FRONT THIGH

■

HAMSTRING

■

UPPER AND LOWER
CALF

■

SIDE

■

CAT/HANGING
(WHOLE BODY)

CAUTION

To protect the spine,
push the pelvis as far
as possible toward the
ground before
beginning step 3.

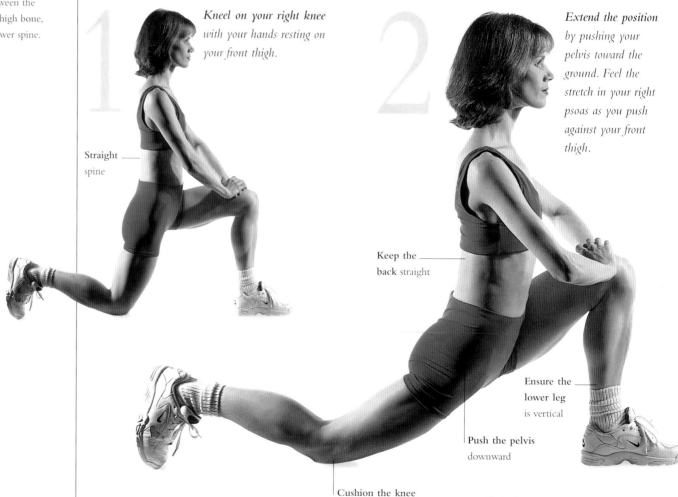

1

Kneel on your right knee
with your hands resting on
your front thigh.

Straight
spine

2

Extend the position
by pushing your
pelvis toward the
ground. Feel the
stretch in your right
psoas as you push
against your front
thigh.

Keep the
back straight

Ensure the
lower leg
is vertical

Push the pelvis
downward

Cushion the knee
with a folded towel
if necessary

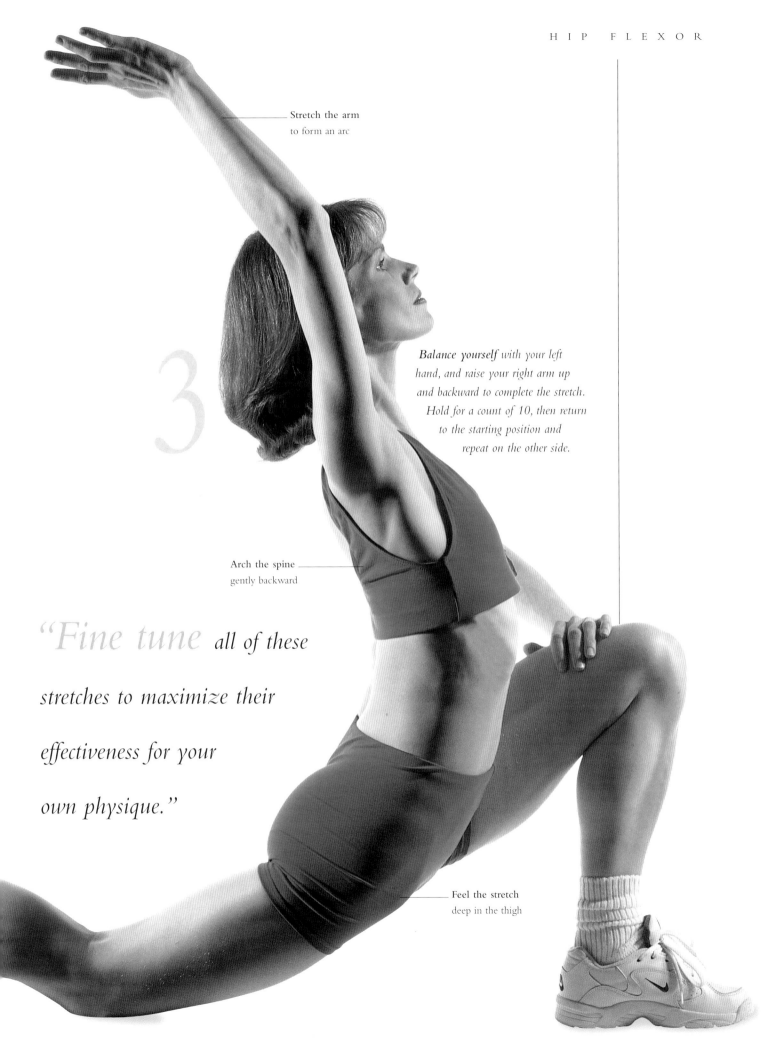

Stretch the arm
to form an arc

3

Balance yourself with your left
hand, and raise your right arm up
and backward to complete the stretch.
Hold for a count of 10, then return
to the starting position and
repeat on the other side.

Arch the spine
gently backward

"*Fine tune* all of these

stretches to maximize their

effectiveness for your

own physique."

Feel the stretch
deep in the thigh

Front Thigh

The rectus femoris is one of the four quadriceps muscles in the front of the thigh. Of the four, it is the only muscle that crosses the hip and knee joints. Any action that involves lifting a straight leg in front of you – kicking a ball for instance – will activate the rectus femoris. If it is tight, it may tilt the pelvis forward, causing problems in the lower back.

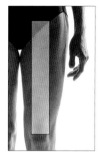

THE RECTUS FEMORIS MUSCLE is located along the front thigh and stretches from the knee to the hip.

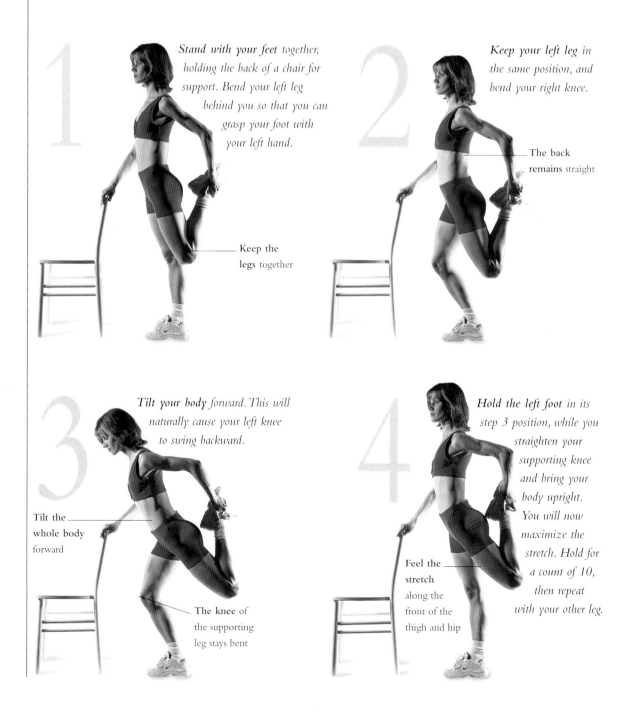

1

Stand with your feet together, *holding the back of a chair for support. Bend your left leg behind you so that you can grasp your foot with your left hand.*

Keep the **legs** together

2

Keep your left leg in the same position, and bend your right knee.

The **back remains** straight

3

Tilt your body forward. This will *naturally cause your left knee to swing backward.*

Tilt the whole body forward

The **knee** of the supporting leg stays bent

4

Hold the left foot in its *step 3 position, while you straighten your supporting knee and bring your body upright. You will now maximize the stretch. Hold for a count of 10, then repeat with your other leg.*

Feel the stretch along the front of the thigh and hip

Hamstrings

The group of muscles in the back of the thigh is collectively known as the hamstrings. They are used to bend the knee and lift the leg behind the body. Tight hamstrings are easily injured, and can also be an indirect cause of back pain.

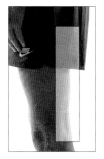

THE HAMSTRINGS originate at the back of the pelvis and attach below the knee.

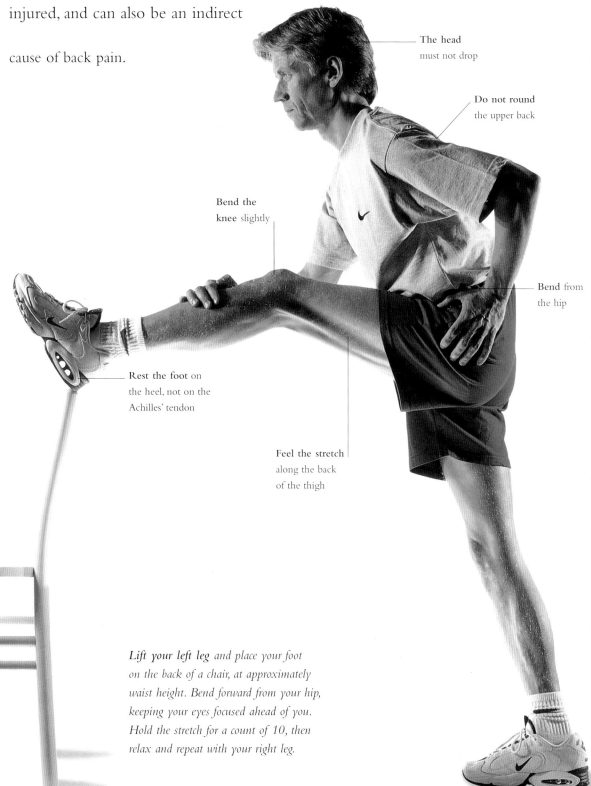

The head must not drop

Do not round the upper back

Bend the knee slightly

Bend from the hip

Rest the foot on the heel, not on the Achilles' tendon

Feel the stretch along the back of the thigh

Lift your left leg and place your foot on the back of a chair, at approximately waist height. Bend forward from your hip, keeping your eyes focused ahead of you. Hold the stretch for a count of 10, then relax and repeat with your right leg.

CAUTION

To avoid stressing the sciatic nerve, keep the raised foot relaxed, the knee slightly bent, and look straight ahead.

85

Upper Calf

The calf has two major muscles: the gastrocnemius and the soleus. The gastrocnemius is the rounded, upper part that provides the powerful push-off used in walking, running and jumping. If tight, it can lead to problems with the Achilles' tendon, to which it is connected, and can distort the alignment of the foot.

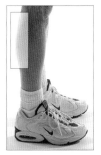

THE GASTROCNEMIUS MUSCLE is in the upper part of the calf. It originates at the femur and inserts at the heel.

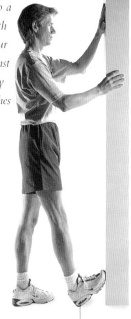

1 *Stand close to a solid wall, with the ball of your right foot against it, so that only your heel touches the ground.*

Lock the heel into the ground

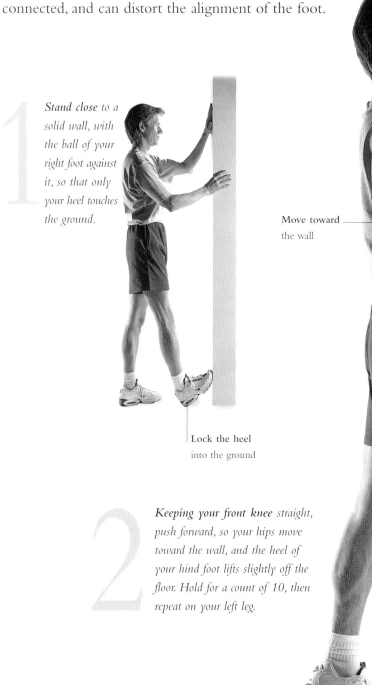

Move toward the wall

2 *Keeping your front knee straight, push forward, so your hips move toward the wall, and the heel of your hind foot lifts slightly off the floor. Hold for a count of 10, then repeat on your left leg.*

Ensure the knee is straight

CAUTION

Move gently from step 1 to step 2, as this technique can generate considerable force.

Lower Calf

The soleus is the broad, flat muscle in the lower part of the calf. Unlike all the other stretches, which involve muscles crossing two joints, the soleus is a one-joint muscle, and only crosses the ankle. One-joint muscles do not usually cause problems, but the soleus needs special attention because it works so closely with the gastrocnemius.

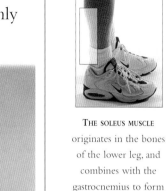

THE SOLEUS MUSCLE originates in the bones of the lower leg, and combines with the gastrocnemius to form the Achilles' tendon.

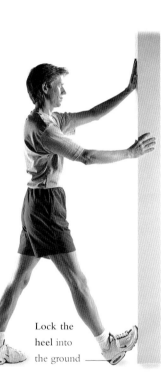

Lock the heel into the ground

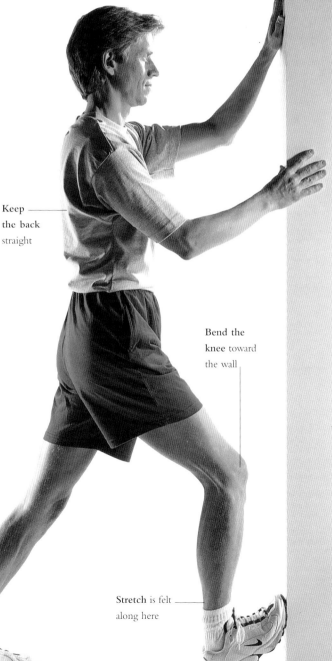

Keep the back straight

Bend the knee toward the wall

Stretch is felt along here

1 *Stand at arm's length from a solid wall. Place the ball of your right foot against it, so that only your heel touches the ground.*

2 *Stretch the lower calf by bending your right knee and pushing it toward the wall. Hold for a count of 10, then repeat with your left leg Follow this stretch by repeating the upper calf stretch opposite.*

87

Side Stretch

This stretch elongates the entire side of the body, from the knee through to the fingertips. Its primary function is to stretch the muscles on the outside of the hip, but this is an all-purpose exercise that also targets the muscles that bend the body to the side and the muscles that lie between the ribs.

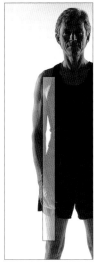

THE TENSOR FASCIAE LATAE and the OBLIQUE ABDOMINAL MUSCLES lie at the side of the body. The INTERCOSTAL MUSCLES lie between the ribs.

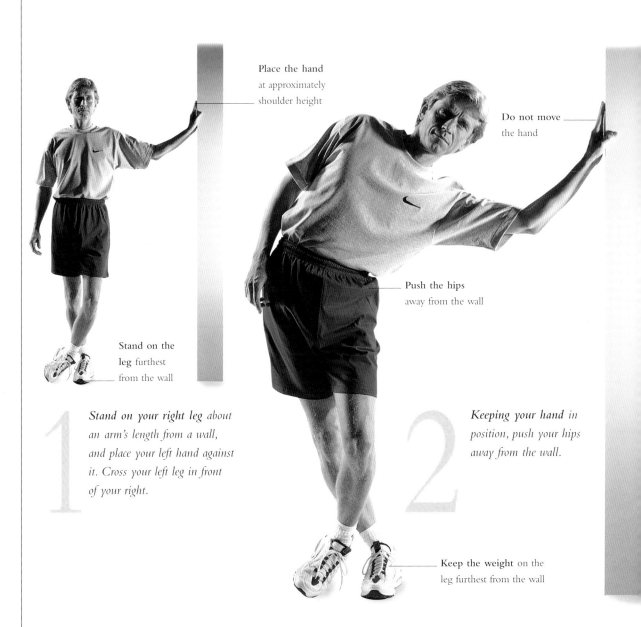

Place the hand at approximately shoulder height

Stand on the leg furthest from the wall

1 *Stand on your right leg about an arm's length from a wall, and place your left hand against it. Cross your left leg in front of your right.*

Do not move the hand

Push the hips away from the wall

2 *Keeping your hand in position, push your hips away from the wall.*

Keep the weight on the leg furthest from the wall

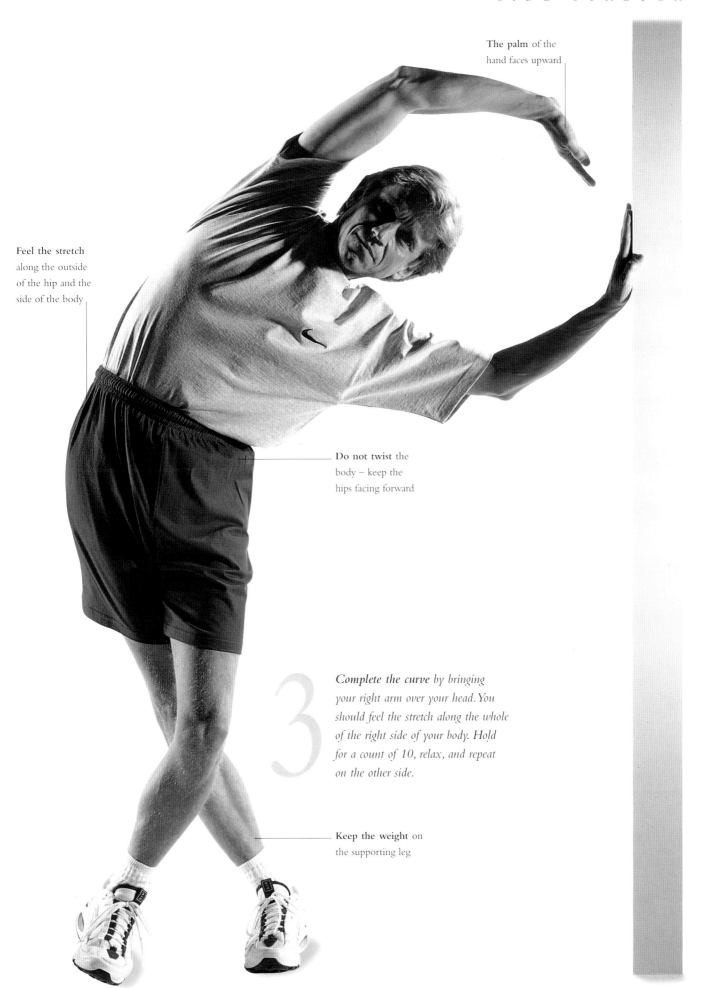

The palm of the
hand faces upward

Feel the stretch
along the outside
of the hip and the
side of the body

Do not twist the
body – keep the
hips facing forward

Complete the curve by bringing
your right arm over your head. You
should feel the stretch along the whole
of the right side of your body. Hold
for a count of 10, relax, and repeat
on the other side.

Keep the weight on
the supporting leg

Cat Stretch

The spine is made up of 24 individual vertebrae held together by muscles, ligaments and discs. A healthy spine relies on mobility between the vertebrae. When this is limited, back problems can arise. The cat stretch is an excellent way to maintain and even increase mobility in the spine, and so guard against back problems.

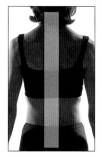

THE VERTEBRAE run all the way down the the back, from the skull to the tail bone.

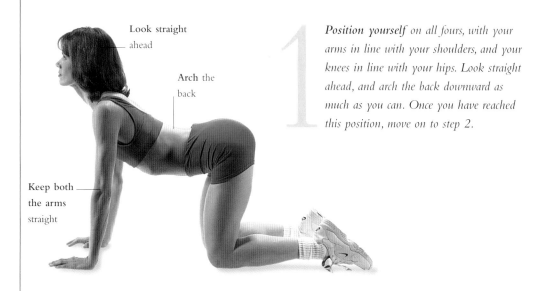

Look straight ahead

Arch the back

Keep both the arms straight

Position yourself on all fours, with your arms in line with your shoulders, and your knees in line with your hips. Look straight ahead, and arch the back downward as much as you can. Once you have reached this position, move on to step 2.

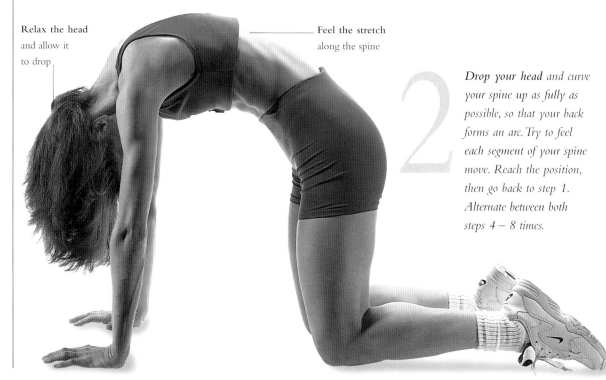

Relax the head and allow it to drop

Feel the stretch along the spine

Drop your head and curve your spine up as fully as possible, so that your back forms an arc. Try to feel each segment of your spine move. Reach the position, then go back to step 1. Alternate between both steps 4 – 8 times.

CAUTION

To avoid neck injury, keep looking straight ahead in step 1.

Hanging Stretch

Ever since man decided to walk upright, the spine has been subject to the negative effects of gravity. The hanging stretch helps to counteract this by providing traction for the spine as well as the shoulder joints. If you do not have a suitable bar (see pages 52 – 53), use a sturdy branch on a tree instead.

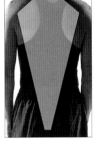

THE SPINAL COLUMN is made up of the vertebrae and encloses the spinal cord, which it protects.

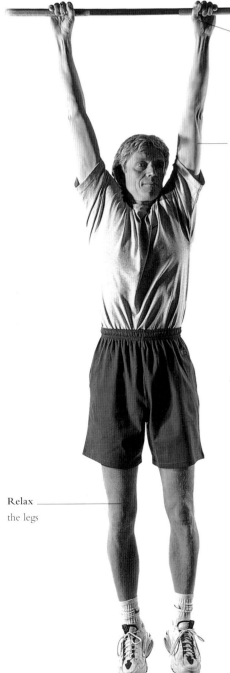

Lock the thumbs around the bar

Check that the body weight falls evenly on both arms

Hang with your arms about shoulder-width apart. Use an overhand grip, with the palms of your hands facing forward (see right). Hold the position for a count of up to 15.

Relax the legs

Overhand grip

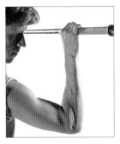

An overhand grip allows you to relax your shoulders. Only the muscles flexing your fingers should be working.

Post-exercise

After you have finished exercising, drink a glass or two of water to replace the fluid you have lost. Eat a high-carbohydrate snack, such as a piece of fruit, to restore your energy.

Do not replace the fat you have just lost!

Glossary

Aerobic Exercise: Low- to moderate-intensity, long-duration exercise, when energy is supplied using oxygen. Aerobic endurance exercise is the only time when fat can be broken down and used directly as the main source of energy.

Amino Acids: Organic compounds necessary in the formation of protein. Essential amino acids cannot be manufactured by the body and must be obtained from food.

Anaerobic Exercise: High-intensity, short-duration exercise that is fuelled by carbohydrates and does not utilize oxygen.

Blood-sugar Level: The concentration of glucose in the blood.

Body Fat: Storage fat that accumulates under the skin.

Calorie: The unit used to indicate the energy value of foods. This energy is used to fuel the body. It is also now measured in joules (1 calorie = 4.19 joules). A "calorie deficit" is when the body uses more calories than the diet provides.

Carbohydrates: The large group of sugars, starches and dietary fibre that contain carbon, hydrogen and oxygen. Carbohydrates are the main source of energy for all body functions, and are needed to process other nutrients. They are formed by all green plants, which use the sun to turn carbon dioxide and water into simple sugar molecules. They can also be made in the body.

Cholesterol: A substance found in liver, egg yolk and some shellfish. It is also made in the human body, mainly in the liver and kidneys. Cholesterol helps to absorb fatty acids and to make vitamin D and various hormones, including the sex hormones, but surplus amounts of it can be dangerous.

Cramp: Prolonged, painful contraction of the muscles, often caused by the imbalance of salts in the body, but more often as a result of fatigue, poor posture or stress.

Diuretic: Tending to increase the flow of urine from the body.

Endorphins: Hormones produced in the brain that have natural pain-relieving qualities. During exercise their production increases, leading to a general sense of wellbeing.

Energy: Needed for the body to function and be active. Measured in calories or joules, and derived from carbohydrates, protein and fat.

Enzymes: Proteins that accelerate biological reactions.

Fat: A substance made up of fatty acids that is found in both animals and plants. It provides a concentrated form of energy and can be stored as body fat.

Glucose: A simple sugar found in certain foods, such as fruit. All other carbohydrates are converted to glucose before the body can use them as its main source of energy. Glucose can be stored in the liver and muscles, as glycogen, then converted to glucose when needed.

Glycogen: The major carbohydrate that is stored in cells. It is an energy source, made from glucose and is stored chiefly in the liver.

Heart Rate: A measure of cardiac activity, usually expressed as the number of beats per minute (BPM).

Hormone: A chemical substance that is released into the bloodstream and carried to specific receptor sites in the body, where it acts to modify their structure or function.

Insulin: Hormone produced by the pancreas, that regulates the body's absorption of carbohydrates.

Lactic Acid: A vital substance in the production of energy, which is recycled when there is sufficient oxygen available. In anaerobic energy production, it builds up in the cells and limits endurance.

Ligament: A tough band of tissue that connects two bones, or holds organs in place.

Metabolism: The collective term for the chemical changes in living cells, by which energy is provided for vital processes like growth and functioning. The "resting metabolic rate" reflects the energy required to keep the body functioning when it is at rest.

Minerals: A group of inorganic substances that occur naturally in the earth's crust and must be included in the diet. They are important in regulating many bodily functions.

Muscles: Tissues with the ability to contract, causing and allowing movement of the joints.

Obesity: A condition characterized by excessive body fat.

Osteoporosis: A condition in which the density of the bones declines, making them brittle and, therefore, prone to fracture.

Protein: A compound of carbon, hydrogen, oxygen and nitrogen that provides the raw materials (amino acids) for growth and repair. Proteins form the structural material of muscles, tissues and organs. In certain circumstances, protein can be converted into glucose and used for energy.

Repetition: A single, completed movement of an exercise.

Resting Metabolic Rate: *See* metabolism.

Set: The name for a group of repetitions.

Target Zone: The heart-rate range for a specific exercise intensity.

Tendons: A tough band of connective tissue that connects muscle to another body part, usually bone, and transmits the force that the muscle exerts.

Vertebrae: The bony segments that, together, make up the spinal column.

Vitamins: Organic substances that neither supply energy nor contribute to body mass, yet have a crucial part to play in almost all body processes.

Index

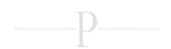

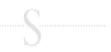

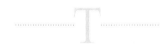

Bibliography

Exercise Physiology; Energy, Nutrition and Human Performance, 4th Edition, McArdle, Katch and Katch, Williams & Wilkins, 1996

Manual of Nutrition, 10th Edition, MAFF, 1995

Gray's Anatomy, 37th Edition, Churchill Livingstone, 1993

Töjning av Muskler, I and II, Evjenth and Hamberg, Alfta Rehab Förlag, 1980

Useful addresses

Chin-up bars:

Polar Electro OY, Professorintie 5, 90440 Kempele, Finland.

Polar Electro Inc, 99 Seaview Blvd, Port Washington, NY 11050, USA
Internet: http://www.polar.fi/

Tunturi, Tunturioyörä Oy, SF 20760, Piispanristi, Finland.
Tel: +358 21 603 111   Fax: +358 21 603 323

Cycle stands:

Tacx Cycletrack, Rijksstraatweg 52, 2241 BW Wassenaar, Netherlands.
Tel: +31(0)70 511 9259   Fax: +31(0)70 511 6411

Cycle-Ops Products, 71 West 11th Street, New York, NY 10011, USA.
Tel: +212 924 6724   E-mail: www.cycle-ops.com

Heart-rate monitors:

Polar, Leisure Systems International Ltd.
Tel: +01926 811 611   E-mail: Isisales@Isi.co.uk
Internet: http://www.polar.fi/sampola/

Acknowledgments

Author's Acknowledgements

I should like to record my gratitude to Torje Eike for advice on the text and constant support, and to Dr Paul Pacy for his generous advice. Torje Eike would like to thank Prof. Patrick Salter of Queen Margaret's College, Edinburgh for instilling in him a life-long interest in anatomy and physiology, and David West, MCSP, for his friendship and professional support over the last decade. We would also like to thank Monica Chakraverty and Robert Ford of Dorling Kindersley for unfailing good humour and valuable advice.

Publisher's Acknowledgements

Dorling Kindersley would like to thank:
Sue Bosanko, Lorna Damms, Nicola Graimes, Nasim Mawji, Jill Scott and Sue Sian. Thanks also to John Woodcock for his illustration work. The following food photography is by Clive Streeter: 44, 46, 48.